SEATTLE'S
MEDIC ONE

SEATTLE'S MEDIC ONE

How We Don't Die

RICHARD RAPPORT, MD

THE
History
PRESS

Published by The History Press
Charleston, SC
www.historypress.com

First published 2019

Manufactured in the United States

ISBN 9781467143608

Library of Congress Control Number: 2019939729

Seattle's Medic One: How We Don't Die *is a fascinating history of the emergence and resounding success of pre-hospital care provided by paramedics. Before these programs existed, many people with a cardiac arrest or major injuries simply died in place before they could get to a hospital. At a time when American health care is challenged by cost, quality and access, the book shines light on how health system innovations built on an ethic of placing patient welfare above the protection of physicians' professional turf can vastly improve outcomes.*
—*Scott Barnhart, MD, former medical director, Harborview Medical Center*

Rick Rapport's excellent recounting of the development of Seattle's first-rate emergency medical system and the remarkable leadership of a few strong minded individuals who drove this forward for decades reminds readers that with conviction, a clear vision, and not taking no for an answer, much can be done to create solutions that have enduring and in this case life-saving, results. More personally, when I was Deputy Mayor of Seattle, I had a chance to encounter Michael Copass on a couple of issues related to the fire department and Medic One. Let's just say I have rarely met someone who was so forceful and yet soft-spoken. Chief Vickery's reputation is legendary as well and lives on in the city. I am grateful to Rick Rapport for capturing this era and aspect of Seattle's history.
—*Maud Daudon, former Seattle deputy mayor and past president/CEO of the Seattle Metropolitan Chamber of Commerce*

If you have a heart, you will be riveted by this account of how we have all come to benefit from pre-hospital emergency services and transportation. Dr. Rapport tells a compelling story of collaboration, innovation, bold personalities, and the power of place. Dramas we know about, like the Oso mudslide, part of a vivid in-depth tribute to medical practitioners, emergency responders, leaders, and dreamers. The story of how this community, with the ethic of "helping anyone no matter what," continually reinvents itself.
—*Lou Oma Durand, executive director, Washington State Department of Services for the Blind*

An engaging account of the early years of Seattle's world-famous Medic One program and its remarkable creators, Drs. Leonard Cobb, Michael Copass and Seattle Fire Department chief Gordon Vickery.
—*Mickey Eisenberg, MD, PhD, associate medical director, King County Emergency Services, and author of* Life in the Balance

Rapport, a Seattle neurosurgeon who has seen it all while working at Harborview in Seattle for more than forty years, tells the story of Medic One from its beginning as an idea in Dr. Leonard Cobb's head, to its evolution as a model for Emergency Medical Services for the rest of the United States and the world. His fascinating story is one of personalities and characters who overcome politics and medical barriers to create a practical model that has saved hundreds of thousands of lives.
—Michael M.E. Johns, MD, dean emeritus, Johns Hopkins School of Medicine, and former chancellor, Emory University

A fascinating read of an absolutely compelling story that I had never thought to wonder about—the invention of a practice that is such a mainstay now, it's nearly impossible to imagine our society functioning without it.
—Lynn Shelton, film actress, writer and director

Dr. Richard Rapport has written a riveting history of Medic One, turning what could be a dry subject into a saga. He tells the compelling, and often intersecting, personal stories of those who developed it (country doctors, researchers, paramedics and ER docs) and shows how their response both to advances in medicine and to real emergencies in areas of limited resources, built the emergency services that save countless lives every day. It's an absolutely fascinating read.
—Emily Warn, founding editor of poetryfoundation.org

In Memory of Arthur A. Ward Jr., MD

Out of this nettle, danger, we pluck this flower, safety.
—William Shakespeare

I can think of no more stirring symbol of man's humanity
to man than a fire truck.
—Kurt Vonnegut

CONTENTS

ACKNOWLEDGEMENTS

I would not have been able to record this history of Medic One without the enormous help and support of dozens of people. First among these are Lenard Cobb, Michael and Lucy Copass, Nancy Tiederman, A.D. Vickery, Ann Henry, and Cindy Button. In alphabetical order, others whom I interviewed, corresponded with, or who sent me materials and advice are:

Jennifer Adgey, Sam Arbabi, Scott Barnhart, Abe Bergman, Eileen Bulger, David Carlbom, Randy Curtis, Richard DeFaccio, Jerry Ehler, Mickie Eisenberg, Dave Eschenbach, Kathy Fair, Roy Farrell, John Fisk, Pat Fleet, Hugh Foy, Laura Grimstad, Len Hudson, Kathleen Jobe, Wanda Johanson, Gregory Jurcovich, Aaron Katz, Ken Linnau, Liz MacNamara, Ron Maier, Sam Mandell, Eunice Marchbank, Chris Martin, Janet Marvin, Steven Mitchell, Anne Newcombe, Graham Nichol, Michael Oreskovich, Carol Ostrom, Ruth Payne, Jim Pridgeon, Jeffrey Riddell, Fred Rivara, Michael Sayre, Mitch Schlosser, Jamie Shandrow, Katrina Soderstrom, Susan Stern, Scott Symons, Al Tourangeau, Wes Uhlman, Robin Walker, Marvin Wayne, Roy Waugh, Janett Wingett, Mike Ylenni.

To all of these people, my sincere thanks. There were others who, in passing, sometimes remembered or corroborated parts of the story, and even if they are unrecorded here, they contributed.

For many years, I have relied on guidance from my wonderful agent, Jessica Papin of the Dystel, Goderich & Bourret Literary Agency. Laurie Krill both saw the value of the work when she acquired it for The History Press and then managed production of the manuscript.

INTRODUCTION

Eldon Holmes died early in the morning on February 29, 1972.[1] His wife heard a loud crash when he fell over purple-faced because his heart had unaccountably stopped beating. Her call to 911 at 7:14 a.m. produced a Seattle Fire Department engine at their apartment by 7:16, and one of the brand-new Medic One rigs a minute later. The paramedics found a middle-aged man on the floor not breathing and pulseless.

Even a few years earlier, Mr. Holmes would have been pronounced dead in his apartment. The last thing he remembered of that Tuesday morning, the final leap year day in February, he was drinking coffee in his kitchen. But thanks to the medics who promptly put a breathing tube into his trachea and shocked his heart back to a normal rhythm, a few weeks later he walked out of the hospital.

In Seattle and all over Western Washington, it is now even more difficult to die at the scene of a cardiac arrest or major trauma than it was forty-five years ago. The paramedics won't let you.

From after World War II until Lyndon Johnson signed Medicare/Medicaid into law on July 30, 1965, the emergency care provided by hospitals, doctors, and nurses hadn't changed much since Abraham Flexner published his paradigm-changing report in 1910. In most hospitals, an emergency room was just that, a big room full of acutely ill people, some sitting up, some lying on gurneys divided into almost individual spaces. Patients might go—or be taken by ambulance—to a private hospital if they had means, but the ER itself was similar everywhere in America.

Sick and injured patients either sat expectantly in a reception area or lay in curtained-off cubicles waiting until a junior house officer or a nurse got around to asking what was wrong, taking their vital signs, and examining them. Then they waited some more until a clerk appeared to find out if they had insurance, cash—or nothing. All of these activities were seldom hurried because, in truth, there wasn't a lot to be done for them.

Almost all doctors and nurses then considered it a part of their professional obligation to provide care to poor, sick, and injured patients when they showed up for treatment regardless of their ability to pay. My father, a thoracic surgeon, claimed that at the first monthly meeting of his County Medical Society a dozen years before Medicare, the treasurer reported a total cost for treating unfunded patients admitted to that county hospital emergency room for the previous twelve months. The society president then added 2 percent for inflation and assessed each member an equal portion of the total to provide care for all of the patients anticipated in the ER during the coming year who would be unable to pay. The physicians each absorbed the loss of their professional fees in that setting as a responsibility.

Even so, only very basic techniques were available for diagnosing and treating the sick people who managed to get to a hospital in 1953. An intern on duty in the ER might have an x-ray taken, order an EKG or a blood count, sew up a wound, set a fracture, or treat an infection. The first antibiotics had then been available for little more than a decade, and bacteria had not yet acquired resistance. If the intern suspected appendicitis, he (there were few female doctors then) might consult a senior resident or attending, expecting that patient would undergo an exploratory laparotomy in the OR. The thinking then was that if you didn't explore a few normal bellies you were missing a lot of appendicitis.

There were no CT scans, no MRIs, no ultrasound, no sophisticated angiography, no minimally invasive operations, no internal fixation of fractures, no cardioversion, and no CPR. There were a few effective drugs, most of them cheap, only relatively simple lab tests, and nothing but the local ambulance to get very sick people to the hospital in the first place. If the patient lacked breath and a pulse when the ambulance arrived to pick him or her up, the driver stopped in the ER only long enough for a doctor to pronounce the patient dead; the vehicle turned into a hearse and went straight to the morgue. There were few lawsuits but lots of room for improvement

And then things quickly began to change.

By the 1960s, new treatments and technologies had sprung into use simultaneously. Bernard Lown and colleagues at the Harvard Medical School first perfected equipment that combined cardioversion and defibrillation in 1959. In the early 1960s, portable DC units became available to reignite stalled hearts and to convert abnormal electrical rhythms to normal beats efficiently, without opening the chest or inserting a needle into the heart itself. Better drugs to treat these cardiac abnormalities arrived on emergency room shelves, and CPR was becoming standard. Over the space of a very few years, doctors suddenly had a lot more ammunition to fight disease and injury, but it was all stored on shelves and in drawers at emergency rooms, or in the Central Supply Departments.

Onto this stage stepped Frank Pantridge, an Irish cardiology consultant at the Royal Victoria Hospital in Belfast, professor at Queens University, and former lieutenant in the British Army Medical Corps during World War II. Dr. Pantridge knew what it meant to be sick. Not only did he have diphtheria as a medical student in 1935, but an astute physician also discovered that Pantridge's illness was complicated by heart block, a combination often fatal. Because of this, his graduation was delayed until about the time war was declared in 1939. Clutching his new medical degree, Dr. Pantridge enlisted in the British army and in 1940 sailed into the heat, smell, and vicious conflict of Southeast Asia.

Following the fall of Singapore in 1942, Pantridge was a Japanese prisoner of war and, along with others condemned to slave labor, spent his captivity building the Burma Railroad. Of the 1,600 British soldiers incarcerated with him at a camp near the kampong called Nikki, in Thailand close to the Burmese border, only 182 remained alive at the end of the ordeal. Pantridge himself barely survived the severe thiamine deficiency and beriberi he contracted because of starvation.[2]

But he did survive to train as a cardiologist, and by 1965 in Belfast, the technologies then emerging convinced Pantridge that for many patients with cardiac arrest and arrhythmias getting to the emergency room was already too late. So, he devised a way to take the ER to them and collected encouraging results.

Based on treatment of more than three hundred people in the field, Pantridge and his house officers John Geddes and Jennifer Adgey published their data in two papers in *The Lancet*, one of the premier medical journals in the world. The first described pre-hospital care of myocardial infarction and the second prognosis following associated ventricular fibrillation.[3] For the first time, patients began to survive cardiac arrest at the place where their hearts had stopped working.

In Seattle, Dr. Leonard Cobb read the papers.

As a young cardiologist, Len Cobb had come in 1957 to the University of Washington faculty and worked mainly at the county hospital, Harborview. By 1963, he was the director of the Harborview Division of Cardiology. He exemplified the academic physician scientist and teacher of that era and quickly understood that the earlier treatment pioneered in Belfast increased possibilities for saving lives, and maybe increased those odds greatly. He also was a savvy enough pragmatist to know that a good idea is only as exceptional as its proof. There are always a lot of good ideas floating around an academic medical center competing both for attention and funding. Len Cobb quietly and systematically went in search of both.

He needed help, and his first ally wasn't a doctor. Sitting in his downtown office in 1968 beginning to ponder his budget for the upcoming year, Seattle Fire Chief Gordon Vickery had a call from Cobb, who knew of the chief only by reputation. Vickery had come up through the fire department ranks. He was strong-willed, politically astute, dedicated to the citizens he served, and a person to be taken seriously. In 1972, after the mayor appointed Mr. Vickery superintendent of the then troubled Seattle City Light, longtime newspaper columnist for both major Seattle papers Emmett Watson wrote that Vickery's "controversial impact had to be measured on the Richter Scale."[4] However, as fire chief, Vickery was enormously popular, and when Len Cobb initially called him to discuss pre-hospital emergency care, he also clearly saw the possibilities.

His budget was one of them. By late 1969, the Seattle economic decline eventually known as the "Boeing Bust" had begun, and competing forces were after every cent that could be squeezed from the city budget. In addition, because of improved building codes, the practical use of home smoke alarms, better communications, and faster response times, fire crews departed their stations less frequently to actually fight big city fires. More and more calls to the firehouses concerned non-fire incidents, but the firefighters' wages still had to be paid—at a time when they were vulnerable to cuts. So, when Chief Vickery heard from Dr. Cobb that the fire department might have a much-expanded role in providing treatment to victims of cardiac events before getting them to the emergency room, he had motivation to support the idea.

And support it Gordon Vickery did. The chief initially had some selling to do, convincing Mayor Wes Uhlman, the Seattle City Council, and the closed family of the firefighters' rank and file (as well as their union) to fund pre-hospital medical care. Eventually, hundreds of young men and women without medical school educations learned to do expertly in the field some of the same things doctors do in hospitals, and do them very quickly and well. The ambitious firefighters who became the early paramedics are another major reason that Medic One succeeded in Seattle.

Cobb and Vickery soon discovered another collaborator in the director of a then still basic Harborview Emergency Room. For the next thirty-five years, the first thing anyone saw when they walked by the nurses' station and into the primitive workroom just inside the double doors opening into the old Harborview ER was the balding head, black-rimmed glasses, and stocky body of Dr. Michael K. Copass.

For medical students, interns, and junior residents, this sight was at once both reassuring and terrifying. Reassuring because the students and house officers all understood that Dr. Copass was there to make absolutely certain that all patients, no matter what was wrong with them, where they came from, what shade of skin they had, what kind of insurance they had or didn't, or what language they spoke, were cared for perfectly.

That was also exactly what terrified the younger staff.

In the new Emergency Department later built on the north end of the hospital, Dr. Copass stood at the center work island inside a glassed-in forty-by-forty-foot square called "the fish bowl" wearing khaki pants, a white shirt with his sleeves rolled up a little, and a tie. A few years later, he added a bandolier arrangement over one shoulder weighed down by a radiophone, several pagers, and a few other tools of his one-man trade. He seldom smiled or looked directly at the people he was talking to as the disarray of a big-city trauma center swirled around him. Computers, cellphones, CT scanners, MRI machines, digital angiograms, and modern ventilators were still stacks of engineering drawings on the design desks of the EMI Corporation, Baxter, Siemens, Boston Scientific, Medtronic, and their successors. What happened to the patients brought to the ER at Harborview Medical Center in those days was entirely determined and supervised by Dr. Copass.

While the junior house staff began to evaluate the broken, intoxicated, infected, and sometimes comatose or dying patients hauled in from around Seattle, aided and advised by various nurses, senior residents, and faculty members, Mike Copass was the person who directed traffic. He decided. While he was tolerant of a lack of knowledge and even uncertainty on the part of the young house staff, medical students, and nurses he supervised, he was absolutely intolerant of intolerance. That is, every patient was to be treated as an important human being. God help the person who ever forgot that first principle, because no one ever forgot it twice.

The last participant in this story of Medic One's success occupied a general practice office in the middle of Washington State. William Henry, MD, was the only doctor in the small town of Twisp in the Methow Valley, a subalpine region in the Cascade Range of Central Washington. Bill Henry, his pregnant wife, Ann, and their two young children had arrived at this outpost in 1960 following his discharge from the U.S. Navy. He hung up a sign, opened his office on Glover Street, hired a nurse, then a receptionist, and Ann Henry paid the bills. Twisp had a new GP.

Such a straightforward undertaking was possible in 1960, but it wasn't easy. The closest hospital was in Brewster, fifty miles down the Methow River. Bill Henry was an old-fashioned generalist, and he took care of almost everything himself. He made rounds and operated at the Brewster hospital, then saw every kind of medical and traumatic emergency either in his office, the patient's home, or where they had fallen. He was on call every minute he was in town and also had to contend with the fact that there was a bar next door to his office. This unfortunate geography ensured that some of the loggers, ranchers, and farmers, as well as any rowdies who got drunk, fought, and injured themselves or each other had only to crawl or be dragged a few feet to Doc Henry's office to get patched up.[5]

But he couldn't patch up everything, of course, and over time, he began to lament that there was no easy (much less safe or reliable) way to transport critically ill patients out of the valley to bigger, better-equipped hospitals where there were ICUs and specialists. Doc Henry tried to invent several solutions to this dilemma, and he finally found one after Cobb, Copass, Vickery, and the firefighters first stationed at Harborview in Seattle put Medic One and later Airlift NW into operation.

This book describes, in part, a story of what early in his career Bill Henry called "The Henry Fake Factor." He meant that if fate delivered a patient to him with an illness that he didn't understand well and couldn't really treat effectively where he was, and if there was no way to transfer that person to a bigger center in time, it was Doc Henry or nothing. So, he tried to do what he could and called that faking it. After Medic One, Airlift, and then the statewide emergency transfer system that Bill Henry helped to organize, he and the hundreds of other small community general practitioners located in hamlets around the Pacific Northwest could safely and efficiently move people to the higher levels of care required.

Chance brought all of these people together at a time when the technology was ripening, the fire department was diversifying, the emergency room was morphing into the emergency department, and the West Coast spirit of adventure and—perhaps more importantly—cooperation, came together to build Medic One in Seattle during those years when similar undertakings often faltered elsewhere.

At the same time, all new ventures are accompanied by unintended consequences. One of the side effects of the paramedics' technical success at saving lives is that some patients delivered to emergency departments with a heartbeat and oxygenated blood really had died at the scene. But no one can know that until specialized physicians collect sophisticated imaging as well as laboratory data and, then, along with experienced nurses, examine these sick and injured people again and again over time. To tell this part of the story in a coherent way while at the same time protecting identities of patients, I have changed names and details in the chapter titled "Some Stages of Instability."

1

WHAT IS DEAD?

What people mean by the term *dead* seems as if it should be simple. But the word has always had cultural as well as physiologic interpretations, and what dead means hasn't always been certain in either context. In addition, the legal definition of death has changed over time and place, and perhaps it is still changing. Like many words, it depends upon where the dead person is and who's speaking for the corpse. It begins anywhere: a heart attack in the workshop, a fall down the basement stairs, a stroke in the garden, or a car crash on the way to the grocery store. Suddenly, the veiled idea that creeps to consciousness in that shadowy moment just before sleep—the alarmed realization that life is, after all, perilous and short—might be a reality right now.

In today's American society, paramedics arrive, often while the 911 dispatcher is still on the phone, and efficiently take charge. They are young, strong, and highly trained. They know how to do what must be done. They push in needles, start IVs, inject drugs, insert tubes into lungs, bladders, and sometimes into the chest or trachea itself. If the heartbeat is absent or irregular, if breathing is labored, they begin resuscitation, forcing back the neck to open the airway for intubation, while pumping sturdily on the sternum, occasionally breaking a rib or deflating a lung.

Intubation was an initial roadblock to the whole idea of paramedics, and in the early years, many doctors and medical organizations vigorously opposed allowing anyone but doctors and specially trained nurse anesthetists to intubate people. When patients aren't breathing or have a compromised airway, salvation comes to them in the form of a slightly curved, flexible plastic tube inserted into the windpipe. Endotracheal tubes are cuffed at the end with an inflatable balloon to seal the trachea, both ensuring inflation of the lungs with oxygen and preventing aspiration of fluids. This procedure requires that the patient's neck be extended and an instrument called a laryngoscope inserted into the mouth, depressing the tongue so that the vocal cords are seen clearly. Seeing the cords ensures that the tube is positioned into the trachea and not the esophagus that connects the back of the throat to the stomach. Anyone intubating a patient must not only be skilled at these tasks but also able to recognize any of the several things that can go wrong in the process.

Once paramedics have intubated a person found down because of a cardiac event, they often can shock an unreliably contracting heart, or one not beating at all, back to regularity. If the patient might have a broken neck, first responders ease the back of a rigid collar around behind the spine and then secure the front half that fits under the chin, tape the head to a board, turn on the lights and siren, then speed to the nearest hospital. When vital signs become unstable on the way, they resuscitate the patient right in the back of their portable emergency department by giving intravenous drugs, fluids, and—sometimes—ongoing CPR.

In the emergency department of a Level 1 Trauma Center, a patient who has been found down immediately has a CT scan from the top of the head to the bottom of the pelvis, and then the ED staff starts to figure out what happened. Limbs askew in non-anatomical alignment, swollen, bruised, or bleeding are x-rayed. When fractures are discovered, they are immobilized until a more permanent fix can be arranged. An anesthesiologist stabs a needle into the radial artery at the wrist, and some of the blood that spurts out is collected in special vacuum tubes with color-coded tops and sent to the lab. Nurses fill more openings with catheters, tubes, and transducers. Technicians come and go with specialized equipment. Interns call the paging operator looking for more senior house officers and consultants. Still, the patient has not moved or spoken or understood.

The gathering of friends and family has grown larger by the time the patient arrives in the ICU. A nurse helps maneuver the gurney into a small room containing a single bed, a console of electronic monitors, suction, and outlets for gases. The anesthesiologist who has come with the patient, squeezing oxygen out of a black rubber Ambu bag into flaccid lungs, connects the endotracheal tube to a ventilator at the bedside. The machine puffs, its slender jointed arm arched over the bed, holding up the hoses that come off the mechanical box, blinking with settings and plugged into the tube now connecting the body with oxygen and respiration.

Life's basic assumptions have vanished; now the patient *requires* the machines. A few hours have passed since it all began, proceedings that lead either to recovery or migration out of life.

But this sequence of events hasn't always been the case.

Determining the end of being isn't a problem for the unconscious patient. It's a problem for everyone else. Defining the moment of death is an ancient puzzle, although the first hominids probably had less trouble deciding who of their fellows was not alive than modern people, plugged into cellphones or other devices and beeping with technology. When australopithecines found a motionless body pierced, broken, or mangled, they no doubt assumed that life was gone and began to look around anxiously to discover the reason so that they could avoid the same harm themselves. As clever people made nosologies describing states of being unwell, the way out of life became more complex. Bambuti (Mbuti) Pygmies of the Congo, for example, describe "various degrees of illness by saying that someone is hot, with fever, dead, completely or absolutely dead and, finally, dead forever."[6] For them, only this final state is irrevocable.

The cultural determinants defining death for people with holistic and spiritual views of the world are as real to them as the physiological ones are to those who collect data. A recent example in Seattle began when several buddies of a twenty-year-old Ethiopian man convinced him that it really didn't matter whether or not he had ever driven a 500cc motorcycle before, he certainly could do it. And he could drive it, at sixty miles an hour without a helmet right into a cement wall. He was, in fact, dead at the scene, but the paramedics didn't know that. So they intubated him, shocked his heart back to a recognizable rhythm, poured in IV fluids, and brought him to the ED at Harborview Medical Center. Shortly after admission, a blood flow study revealed that his intracranial pressure exceeded the ability of his heart and arteries to push blood into his brain, and he soon was pronounced brain dead. But by then, he was on a ventilator and maximal life support. When the family and friends were given the news that he was brain dead, they were astonished. "How can he be dead? His heart is beating, and he is still breathing. Of course he isn't dead." It was only after four more days when his heart finally stopped that they abandoned hope.

Gas exchange and the oxygenation of hemoglobin were poorly understood until the late eighteenth century. Although as early as two hundred years after Christ there was a suspicion that life is somehow related to breath when Galen taught that respiration cooled the heart, details were lacking. Eventually, scientists noticed that breathing kept mammals alive. But even as late as 1669, Samuel Pepys claimed in his diary that physicians were mystified by respiration.[7] While they realized that it was essential, he wrote, they had no idea what it actually was for or how it worked. To forestall mistakes, friends sometimes held mirrors in front of the nose and mouth of those suspected of being dead in an effort to expose the exhaust of a still faintly moving breath. Indeed, the abundant literature and folklore of the seventeenth and eighteenth centuries surrounding premature interment led not only to the rite of *conclamatio*—loudly calling the dead person's name three times—but also testator's precautions, which were legal rather than sacramental. While the church incorporated customs for exhibition of the body—loud noises, exposure of the face, and a waiting period before burial—in an effort to ensure the corpse was dead forever, even so a body occasionally sat up while being measured for its shroud and coffin.

Because of fear and uncertainty, wills often included precautions directing survivors to wait several days, not touching the corpse at all and especially not cutting it open, before burial. Sometimes, family members were instructed to scratch the feet of the corpse after a few days, or less specifically, to use "all modern methods" to ensure that the body was not sealed up prematurely. In some instances, the terror of being buried alive caused people to admonish that bells be attached to the limbs of their corpses, hoping to announce movements. The details of how this would work after interment when the mourners had gone home were not addressed, a situation analogous in its simplicity to the modern wish to freeze bodies (or sometimes simply heads) after death, preserving them until a cure for their demise might be discovered.

Physicians rarely certified death and were reluctant to get involved in burial, both because they feared being wrong and because they wished to distance themselves from the failure of their own treatments. Today's advance directives, which instruct physicians on how to provide care during a final illness, were therefore preceded by documents just as carefully crafted that describe how to treat a body when death was merely presumed.

In 1628, William Harvey published *De Motu Cordis*, his treatise explaining the circulation of the blood. Though initially vilified by his colleagues for challenging the inviolable truths of Galen (who actually had put an end to much medical investigation and new learning for centuries), Harvey understood heartbeat and circulation of blood through vessels because he ignored that dogma and made his own observations. For the next three centuries, until the late 1960s, the presence of pulse and respiration alone defined a living being.

In 1968, a research group at Harvard developed criteria to determine when a person was dead, not by cessation of breathing or circulation, but by death of the brain.[8] Because today we equate personhood with mind and mind with brain, death of the brain seems the best way to define death of the person. Initially, these criteria were cumbersome and overly complex, but eventually they were refined, simplified, and accepted not only by health care professionals but, more importantly, by the public and the courts as well. Since the adoption of the Uniform Definition of Death Act in 1978, brain death is widely accepted in America (and also in Europe) as the death of a person.

This absence of brain activity supplanted the absence of heartbeat as defining death at the same moment Bernard Lown and colleagues developed a method to reignite a not-beating heart, or to regularize one that was beating erratically. Lown wasn't the first person to shock a stilled heart into life, and the first patients weren't even humans, they were hens. In 1775, Peter Abildgaard electrocuted the heads of chickens with a primitive battery called a Leyden jar and then resuscitated them with a second blast of electricity across the breast. By the 1950s, researchers in Russia had begun to understand DC cardioversion, but they were well hidden behind the Iron Curtain. On a goodwill trip in 1958, Senator Hubert Humphrey visited the cardiac research lab of Naum Gurvich and later wrote, "There, I saw his successful animal experiments on the reversibility of death, that is, on the revival of 'clinically dead' animals through massive electric shocks."[9]

Lown and his group took the "massive" out of this description and developed a simple and straightforward method for delivering DC shocks to an abnormal heart that worked. Suddenly, someone without a heartbeat was not necessarily dead. But what then did it mean not to have a beating heart?

That is the question Frank Pantridge sought to answer in Belfast. Intensive Care Units had begun to appear in hospitals by the early 1960s, and better survival after heart attacks was being reported. John Geddes, then a registrar at the Royal Vic, found an article published in 1948 noting that half of the patients studied died within an hour of the onset of symptoms of myocardial infarction.[10] The habit in Northern Ireland in the mid-twentieth century was that people with chest pain (or any other pain, for that matter) phoned the local GP for advice. This beleaguered doctor might arrive to have a look after the patient was already cold. Even if the hospital dispatched an ambulance, it could take several hours to show up.

So Pantridge decided to take the coronary care unit to the people.

He had no funding for this project, and few people other than he and his house officer, John Geddes, believed it would work. Eventually, he got a small grant from the British Heart Foundation. Then he found an old ambulance and, with the help of a hospital maintenance engineer, rigged up a portable DC defibrillator, sending a driver, a nurse, and Geddes out into Belfast to shock people back into life.

In the 1967 *Lancet* articles, Frank Pantridge, John Geddes, and Jennifer Adgey reported the data they collected treating 312 patients over fifteen months. Their success brought the emergency room to patients and brought previously dead patients back to life.

This was big news to doctors in America.

2

MOBY PIG

After he read the *Lancet* papers, an enthusiastic Leonard Cobb began to think about how he might bring the sophistication of the Seattle medical community to the ideas Frank Panrtidge had shown at least sometimes worked in Belfast, and to improve on that basic system. Years later, Dr. Cobb remarked that the original methods in Ireland were, "very primitive, so the fact that they saved anybody's life was somewhat of a miracle."[11]

The way to introduce new ideas and strategies into medicine, Cobb knew, was with data. He wanted to be able to demonstrate that pre-hospital care increased the number of lives saved out of the total number of patients at risk. Initially, he was interested in tracking only cardiac events. In other words, he wanted to know the denominator, as researchers studying populations like to say, sometimes just to say something that isn't a number. Even today, at the age of ninety-two, a spry Leonard Cobb is often found in the new Medic One office at the Harborview Medical Center helping organize investigations and analyze data, still seeking better methods for saving the lives of patients who collapse from a quivering or silent heart.

By 1969, the confluence of ideas then flowing together in various branches of medicine, and especially in medical schools and teaching hospitals, enabled a whole prescription pad of new possibilities. Not only were chemical and electrical cardioversion and defibrillation established beyond doubt, the drugs and equipment for doing these procedures had been simplified and compacted. Coronary care units and other intensive techniques were part of routine in-patient treatment at major centers and moving out to larger community hospitals by then. At the same time, newer drugs, more options for emergency treatment, efficient mechanical ventilation, and better emergency room technology rapidly appeared.

As a young academic looking for a career niche, Len Cobb was an ideal, thoughtful scientist to help build a system for taking these emerging medical marvels out of the hospital and directly to patients with severe cardiac emergencies. Born in St. Paul, Minnesota, in 1926 and growing up during the Depression, Cobb had a public education and graduated from high school a little early, at the age of seventeen. In 1943, knowing he would soon be drafted in the midst of World War II, he chose his service and enlisted in the navy, where he trained to be an electronics technician. After he served for two years, learning a good bit about tubes, oscilloscopes, radar and sonar, the war ended. He enrolled as an undergraduate at the University of Minnesota and then went straight into the Minnesota Medical School. From there, his route was peripatetic: an internship at the University of Iowa, junior resident at the University of California, research in Sweden for a year, back to California to finish his internal medicine residency, and then to both Harvard and Stanford as a cardiology fellow. He arrived in Seattle in 1957 to join the UW faculty and soon began attending at what was then called Harborview Hospital.

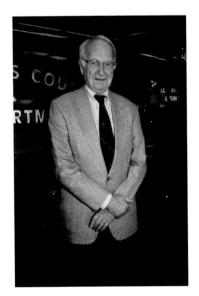

Cobb's grandfather, an old-fashioned country doc working near Grafton, North Dakota, had provided him with a model for how to be a physician. When Cobb was a young child, this grandfather had taken him along to make house calls on farmers and their families. The boy sat in the car or talked to the cows, but he didn't really see the patients unless they wandered over to see him. But his admiration for his grandfather, and the house call experiences, led him to medical school and then to internal medicine.

Physical diagnosis was the one tool a country doctor had early in the twentieth century, and cardiologists especially were trained then to listen intently with their stethoscope to expose the sounds made by

Dr. Leonard Cobb.
Courtesy of Medic One.

30

a diseased heart. Coronary artery angiography done in search of diseased blood vessels, pioneered by André Cournand and Dickinson Richards in the 1940s, wasn't really available to many but them until well after World War II. More modern ultrasound came much later. Until that time, cardiologists bent over and listened to what the chest had to tell them. Then they hoped there was a treatment available for that particular sound.

When Dr. Cobb met Dr. Pantridge remotely through the *Lancet* article, he decided the best way pre-hospital care could be provided to cardiac victims in Seattle was to utilize an existing system capable of hurrying to the scene. That, he reasoned, was the Seattle Fire Department. Doctors would perhaps be able to diagnose and immediately treat cardiac irregularity on the spot, or at least deduce whether or not the patient was suffering a cardiac irregularity or myocardial infarction. What Dr. Cobb then needed was money, a vehicle, and staff, all of which he thought the fire chief could help him acquire. He was right.

Chief Gordon Vickery had a collection of talents.[12] He must have been a capable firefighter to rise in the department as rapidly as he did and a good administrator to pass more senior people. At age forty-three, he was named the youngest fire chief in Seattle's history. But he also was a clever politician and a master publicist. He certainly saw, very early, the value of an expanded role for the fire department in emergency services. He knew well how to make friends in Seattle and King County, and he knew that in part because his way up to where he now stood had not been easy.

Born in 1920 in Ruthton, a tiny agrarian community in Minnesota, Vickery hailed from the same part of the Great Plains as did Len Cobb. He grew up with a father ill with tuberculosis and a mother forced to run a restaurant in the little town on her own. A.D. Vickery, Gordon's son, now also an assistant fire chief in Seattle, recounted, "These were hard times for my father and his sister, both of whom had to work in the restaurant helping to make a meager living. My dad also occasionally worked for his uncle who had a small trucking business (one truck) hauling any cargo they could. The Depression arrived in full swing, and the restaurant closed."

In 1941, their mother moved the family to Snohomish, Washington, because her sister lived there. During the trip, Vickery's father got sicker, and he died soon after they arrived. His mother, now alone with two kids, became a "Rosie the Riveter" during World War II and was known for a dedicated work ethic at Boeing.

Gordon Vickery's first job in Snohomish was with a rural undertaker, because that was the job he got. In those years, the undertaker usually had a vehicle that could also serve as an ambulance, and many morticians did double duty driving to the cemetery by day and to the hospital at night. In fact, when Shepard Ambulance moved from Portland to Seattle in 1922, Frank Shepard had to sign a "non-compete agreement" that he wouldn't open a funeral home. At the same time, local funeral directors found it worth their while to give up the ambulance business. That agreement didn't extend into Snohomish County, so Vickery had early exposure to emergency services, both in various country homes and along the rural roads.

After graduating from high school, he joined the National Guard at the same time the City of Seattle annexed everything up to 145th Street in 1948. A bigger city expanded the Fire Department and created new jobs, some for returning veterans and members of the National Guard. Vickery was one of those National Guardsmen who was hired, and over the next fifteen years he worked his way up through the ranks.

By 1963, the frugal William Fitzgerald had been the Seattle fire chief for exactly a quarter century. A fire station couldn't get a new light bulb unless the burned out one was turned in to the chief's office. Fitzgerald's mission in life was a little different from that of most city executives: to always turn *back* money to the city council at the end of the year. While this largesse resulted in more cash for the city treasury, it also meant that all the equipment was older than Fitzgerald by the time he retired, because there had been no expectant replacement program. In fact, nothing was replaced unless it couldn't be found, stopped running, or completely broke. Chief Fitzgerald had, after all, lived through the Great Depression. For the incoming chief in 1963, a lot of recruit training would be about finding a way to replace sections of hose because they had burst and been repaired so often. It was, as surgeons happening on difficult times in the operating room have been heard to mutter, "like sewing moonbeams to flatus."

When Fitzgerald announced his retirement, there were three final candidates to replace him: two assistant chiefs and Gordon Vickery, only a battalion chief at the time. In that era, there was no large committee, no days of hearings when an important post became vacant. The mayor just named a new fire chief. The assistant chief considered the frontrunner was rumored to have said in a fire station, "I'll tell you what. Tomorrow morning when they announce me as the new chief I'm going to send Vickery so far into the hinterlands that you will never see him again."[13] The next morning, the mayor named Gordon Vickery to the position.

In 1964, at a time when Seattle newspapers had actual reporters on the street rather than on the Internet, Steve Miletich wrote an enthusiastic piece

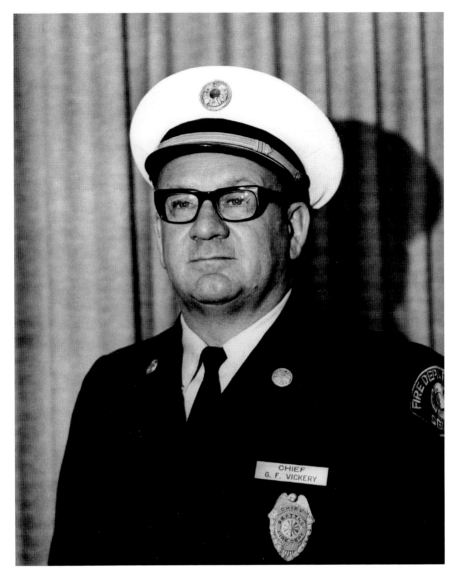

Chief Gordon Vickery, 1970s. *Courtesy of Medic One.*

about the Fire Department's emergency services.[14] His article in the Sunday *Seattle Times* quoted Chief Vickery describing department responses to 1,451 life rescue emergencies the previous year, or about four calls a day. These were the aid car runs. Since his first days as chief, about half a dozen of these dedicated vehicles were part of double houses, meaning a station with both an engine and a ladder company. The *Times* article said Vickery had added, "[L]ife-rescue service is strictly an emergency service. It's not intended for transport such as an ambulance provides." In his brief statement, the chief let the public know when to call for help and also informed the private ambulance companies that he was not out to steal their trade.

Heart attacks, bleeding, and trouble breathing were common causes of calls for help, the newspaper story continued. Of course, those in distress had to reach the department, so Chief Vickery advised learning the phone number, not yet 911—but then a now antiquated five digits preceded by an abbreviated word: MA 2-3344. He ended by saying "Our life-rescue service is an added service beyond what a fire department normally is expected to do. But we're happy to provide it. What better service can you render than saving lives."

Len Cobb later recalled that he had had no selling to do at his first meeting with the fire chief, calling him "an imaginative guy." Vickery was enthusiastic about the plan and eager to help get it moving through the city bureaucracy. Though the aid cars had already been in operation for six years, those firefighters who rode them initially were trained only in advanced first aid, a comparatively modest certificate supervised by the state requiring little medical oversight. Vickery was eager to help build a much more ambitious system.

Of course, Dr. Cobb wasn't the only bright young cardiologist who read the *Lancet*, and doctors in big cities like Miami, Columbus, Pittsburgh, and Los Angeles were also busy trying to design pre-hospital care programs. In some places, the work was cooperative, but often there were competing forces, and in those cases, failure was the rule. Like Seattle, the successful Miami system began operations in 1969. Grants to get started on these ventures were available through the NIH Myocardial Infarction Research Unit, and in 1967, Cobb applied for one but was turned down.

In the fall of 1969, a Seattle Fire Department newsletter announced, "Starting October 14th, ten Seattle Fire Fighters will be assigned to Harborview Hospital [now Harborview Medical Center] on an indefinite detail to commence study preparatory to placing Seattle's first Mobile Coronary Care Unit in service."[15] Funding by the Washington/Alaska Regional Medical Program from the Department of Health, Education, and Welfare was part of Lyndon Johnson's Great Society, and Len Cobb's influence could be felt on the subject of heart attacks. The grant went to the University of Washington with Cobb as the program director, awarding $450,000 over thirty months for salaries, equipment, and drugs. Though each firefighter was then making about $10,000 a year, the grant ensured that the City of Seattle paid nothing more for the ones assigned to Harborview. Newsletter readers learned that about 60 percent of heart attack victims died within one hour of the onset of symptoms and that the majority died "far removed from intensive care units found in modern facilities." Len Cobb was sure that the data he intended to collect would prove that driving the emergency room to the patients rather than waiting for them to appear would save lives.

The actual vehicle the firefighters would first take into the community was a "large, walk-in type van, large enough to stand and work on a patient," and loaded with the usual first aid equipment. But in addition, it carried an EKG machine and a portable DC defibrillator (although at thirty-three pounds, the Physio Control early Life Pak device was really only *almost* portable).

The firefighters immediately christened the unwieldy, underpowered boat of a van with the moniker Moby Pig.[16] It hit the streets on October 13, 1969, and although a lot was expected from this first "super ambulance," it almost immediately bottomed out. The first class of paramedics were all to learn it didn't work very well, not because the idea was unsound but because the first vehicle was. Set on an Oldsmobile motor home chaise, the interior was poorly designed to serve as an emergency response vehicle. It had handled well enough on a three-day journey from Hutchinson, Kansas, where it had been assembled, but that trip was on the interstate. When it arrived in Seattle, the suspension struggled when it bounced up and down the hills, and it was underpowered. Furthermore, Harborview is at the bottom of one hill and the top of another. Moby Pig could go downhill fast enough, though bottoming out all the way, but coming up after leaving HMC it often stalled and died by the time it reached the top of the hill at Broadway. Coming up from downtown, the James Street hill often proved insurmountable.

Still, many firefighters were motivated to become paramedics. Since Vickery had supported Medic One from the start, the program enjoyed popularity, even though there was some early resistance from the conservative rank and file. Fire departments are fraternal and traditional by nature and often reluctant to change.

Certain early paramedics, however, loved both change and opportunity. Dick Shanklin, who graduated in the first class and rode Moby Pig, was one.[17] He was eccentric enough, his colleagues said, to try anything. When a fire broke out on the Ballard ship canal waterfront, the first firefighters on the scene found there was no hydrant. So Shanklin backed the rig down a boat ramp until the three-and-a-half-inch intake was submerged and

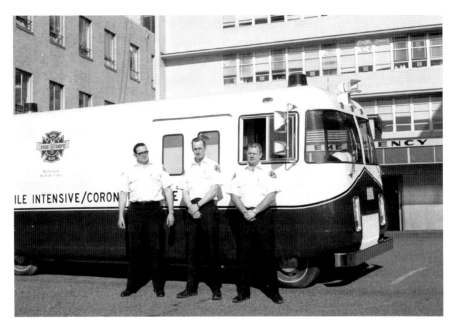

Moby Pig behind Harborview, 1970. (*Left to right*) Paramedics Stan Yantis, Ken Beach, and Jim Dixon. *Courtesy of Seattle Fire Department.*

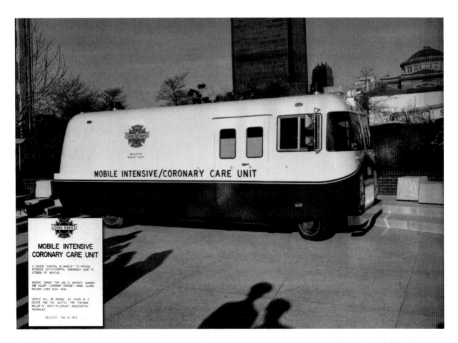

Outside 1970 press conference announcing the beginning of service for original Mobile Intensive Cardiac Unit—Moby Pig. *Courtesy of Seattle Fire Department.*

started pumping water *into*, not out of, the rig. When the tank filled, this worked well enough to quell the blaze. Dick was interested in Medic One because it expanded possibilities for action. There were a lot of smart, at the time mainly high school–educated people, in the fire department who liked challenges and the adrenalin rush necessary to fight fire. Others of them had interests in medicine, so they became paramedics.

However, these first few tentative steps toward effective pre-hospital emergency care depended not so much on specific equipment or structure but rather on cooperation between the fire department, as a part of city government, Dr. Cobb, and the then Harborview Hospital staff. Both Cobb, who brought the idea and necessary background, partnered with the dogged and politically energetic Chief Vickery, were designed to put the project and the community ahead of themselves. What they needed next was the right person to organize and supervise implementation of the program they had developed in their minds.

Fortunately, he was just down the hall.

3

THE ACCIDENTAL ICON

At the time it was called King County Hospital, the original ER at Harborview was eight curtained-off cubicles in a room on the first floor at the south end of the building. To receive the arriving Shepard ambulances, deliveries by the police, or those just able to walk or drag themselves in, the entry to that tiny space opened directly onto a nurses' station where stable patients were registered, triaged, and then waited to be seen by a nurse and a junior house officer. Next, they waited some more while a clerk figured out whether they had insurance, cash—or nothing. Those patients with life-threatening trauma got intubated, ventilated by hand with an Ambu bag, loaded onto the adjacent elevator just large enough by a couple of inches to accommodate a gurney and two residents if they weren't very big, and taken up several floors to the original operating rooms.

That was the whole show.

Beginning in 1973, the first thing chief residents told their juniors and medical students about to start a rotation in the Harborview ER was "don't piss off Dr. Copass." It wasn't that Michael Copass, the newly appointed director of Emergency Services, was unreasonable or quarrelsome (although he once did describe himself to a medicine resident as "short, fat, and angry," winking at a bystander after he said it), but he certainly had his own inviolable view of the world. And this medical and social worldview had evolved from the time he was a little boy growing up on Magnolia Bluff in Seattle.

His story, however, starts not looking out over the Pacific from Seattle's westernmost vantage point but first in Tennessee, Kentucky, Alabama, and Georgia, and after that in East Texas—always among the Baptists.[18] Two families rooted in these deeply southern and border states hybridized to produce Professor Michael Keys Copass; their branches began winding together in the middle of the nineteenth century. His father (christened Mike, not Michael) was a son of the Baptist minister Benjamin Copass, born in central Tennessee the last year of the Civil War. All his life, that grandfather kept in his house the little basket he had used for gathering acorns to grind into the flour that helped keep the family alive. Benjamin Copass married Cornelia Jane Keys, merging two Southern Baptist families into the line that produced Mike. During the War Between the States, battles to control the iron district of middle Tennessee, vital to the South, had largely destroyed the agrarian culture these families had known for generations. Sherman's march to the sea killed what remained of their communities, especially for the Keys clan.

After Benjamin and his brother Jack graduated from Bethel College, a small seminary school in Kentucky, they escaped for California, where they intended to make their fortunes planting orange groves. When they didn't make much of anything, Benjamin returned to preaching and had churches in several small Texas towns: Waxahachie, Denton, Waco, Cleeburn. Like many nineteenth-century evangelicals, Benjamin Copass was theologically conservative but socially progressive, and he believed scripture demands social justice. He later wrote books about the Old Testament prophets and worked to find sensible solutions to the problems of abolition and women's rights. In 1918, Benjamin became professor of Old Testament interpretation at Southwestern Baptist Theological Seminary in Fort Worth, Texas. He and Cornelia had three children, two girls and the boy they baptized Mike.

"My dad was a bit of a rascal and was sent to the Baptist San Marcos Military Academy," Dr. Copass remembered of his preacher's son father. "He was a good athlete, played football as a 140-pound punt returner, and boxed. He was bright enough to go to Baylor, and was editor of their yearbook, *The Roundup*, of which he was quite proud. Dad met Lucile Dean, my mother, in a Browning poetry class at Baylor." The fact that Dr. Michael Copass had a father named Mike, as well as an aunt Lucy, a mother named Lucy (Dean) Copass, and then married Lucy (Ames) Copass, introduces some difficulty in sorting out these relationships.

After the senior Mike Copass graduated from Baylor, he entered Yale Law School but didn't last there long because he had to work shoveling coal into basement bins to support himself when he might better have been studying. Relatives gave him enough money to get back into law school, this time at the University of Chicago. His older sister, Cloantha (named by her classically inclined father for Chloanthus, a minor character in the *Aeneid*), earned a PhD in English tapestries at the same school. His younger sister, Lucile, had a master's in education, also from the University of Chicago. Cloantha raised both her younger brother and sister because their mother had died in childbirth when Lucile was born. This time, the future Dr. Copass's father managed to make ends meet throughout law school—not by shoveling coal but by writing as a stringer for the *Chicago Tribune* sports page. He graduated and then drifted around the country riding the rails (in boxcars, not Pullmans) looking for a job. When he got to Ellensberg, Washington, he hitched a ride on a potato truck to Seattle, and there he stayed—because it was the last option. He later told his children he loved the climate and the orderliness.

The other root of the family, earlier in time and deeper in the South, grew from David Moore. This legend was Dr. Michael Copass's maternal great-grandfather, a three-hundred-pound horse-and-buggy general practitioner of great goodwill, always known in the family as Granddad but by the sick he tended in Blount County, Alabama, as Old Dr. D. Long before Flexner confirmed that a medical education should be scientific, Dr. Moore had intermittently attended the Emory School of Medicine between the end of the harvest and spring planting, when his labor on the family farm was less required, a respite allowing him to be two hundred miles away in Atlanta for seven or eight months. Later in life, he had to hire a driver to take him on his rural rounds, as he had outgrown his ability to hitch a horse to his buggy and to drive it.

Two of the six children Granddad fathered, David and Joseph, referred to as Uncle D and Uncle Joe, also became doctors, living in Birmingham, Alabama, where they founded the Highlands Clinic. Lucile Dean Copass, Michael's mother, was the daughter of Mary Pearl Moore, Uncle D's daughter. She remembered riding out in the country on a house call with her uncle Joe in North Alabama and rolling morphine pellets for a woman dying of breast cancer they found lying on a straw mattress.

Medical doctors had a value in the family almost as great as those southern state Baptist values that included a personal uprightness and a robust social progressivism.

• • • •

In 1932, when the elder Mike Copass climbed off the potato truck and started looking for work, there was stress in Seattle as there was all over Depression-era America. He got a job as a new lawyer in an established firm and stayed for five years before opening up an office with his friend Charles Hall. These two remained colleagues until 1943, when Mike went to work in the Office of Price Administration. Ultimately, he decided he couldn't stay at the OPA because he thought he was shirking his wartime duty to the country, so he tried to join the army, then the navy, then the air force. Despite one bad eye from iritis, the Thirteenth Army Air Force 365th Bomb Squad finally found him an acceptable recruit, sent him to basic training and then to the Pacific theater, headquartered in Hawaii.

Michael K. Copass was born in 1938, and his sister Nancy came two years later. Their father was soon fighting with the Army Air Corps at Midway and Guadalcanal. Before shipping out, he told his small son, "Take care of your sister." Nancy, like her dad, was found to have iritis, and during these fatherless years, her big brother often took her on the city bus to see one of several different ophthalmologists. As a little girl, she announced

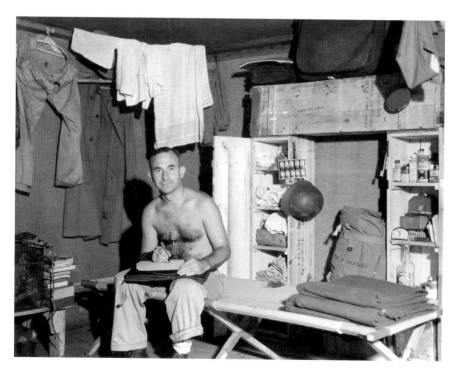

Major Copass in the Pacific theater in 1944. *Courtesy of Nancy Copass Tiederman.*

one day that she wasn't going to see eye doctors anymore. Michael asked her why. "She stopped her toneless whistling and told me that the last guy had dirty fingernails and if he won't care for his own dirty fingernails he won't care for my eyes." For years, Dr. Copass gave this speech to residents and med students about the probity of careful hand-washing and personal appearance. "People do look at you to see if you are well turned out," he lectured to the crowds of often sleep-deprived, unkempt residents and medical students slouched around him in untucked scrubs.

The summers of the war years, the diminished Copass family spent in the Okanagan of British Columbia, at Trepannier Creek. It was in those years Michael Copass developed trouble with his feet. Dr. Roger Anderson, who took care of the family, had insisted that a warm, dry environment, short pants, and days in the sunshine to promote vitamin D production would benefit young Mike's deformity. According to his sister, now Reverend Nancy (Copass) Tiederman, as a young boy he suffered from an unnamed abnormality that required his legs and feet to be casted for several months in 1944.[19] During that time, Michael still remembers Daniel Onion from Kelowna, who perhaps in reply to his name was an awful bully, could jump heroically off the end of a gravel-loading pier and paddle around in Lake Okanagan. In part because of the frail feet, Mike couldn't swim or dive very well, but didn't want Daniel to beat him at anything so he taught himself to leap off that pier the next summer.

In an April 14, 1944 letter sent to Major Mike Copass at the behest of his wife, who was trying to clarify the child's leg and foot ailment, Dr. Anderson explained why she often kept young Michael home from school. He had learned to play baseball in the walking casts that he wore for several years, as he recalled it. He couldn't run after those who bullied him, but when the casts finally came off, he remembered who they were. "In high school, I took aim at everyone who had offended me and challenged them to warfare. I did OK and didn't disgrace myself, because if I came home looking bad my dad had his rule; don't come home looking bad unless the other guy looks worse."

When their father had finally returned home from war, the two children were still in British Columbia with their mother, and Nancy (even then a very direct person) asked him if he was *really* her father. In fact, the return of the long absent male parent disrupted the smoothly running, although a little bit penurious, family life of the mother and two kids. His son later said, "I was truly afraid of him, I think, because he suddenly appeared and broke up this happy little unit. He didn't make suggestions, he gave orders." He'd

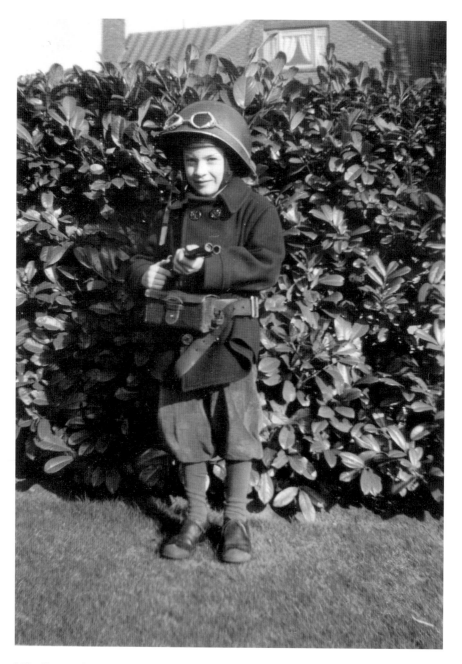

Mike Copass, about six, dressed as a World War II–era soldier. *Courtesy of Nancy Copass Tiederman.*

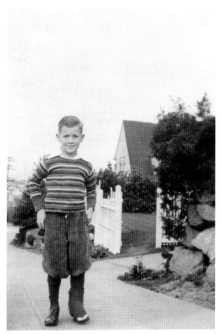 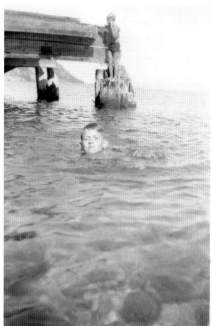

Left: Mike in cast, age six. *Courtesy of Nancy Copass Tiederman.*

Right: Mike swiming in Lake Okanoggen. Danial Onion on the pier, 1944. *Courtesy of Nancy Copass Tiederman.*

been a major in the wartime army and was used to giving orders. The father, like many soldiers returning from World War II, had been living a male life, was used to the orderly structure of the army and was a product of the time when men were assumed to be the head of the household. He also had deeply held social beliefs, as much as they might have evolved over the past seventy-five years. Happy to be home, Major Copass simply assumed that he would resume being in charge, but the rest of the family was not so sure.

The parents had argued about manliness, especially after the returned soldier discovered that his wife had sent their boy to ballet lessons at Mary Ann Wells School of the Dance during the war, as another method for strengthening his frail feet. The unabashed Nancy remembers asking her mother at one point, "Oh, why don't you just divorce him?" The idea of divorce, however, would certainly never have occurred to her mother or father, just as the spectacle of Dr. Michael Copass in tights would have dumbfounded generations of his UW medical students, residents, and colleagues.

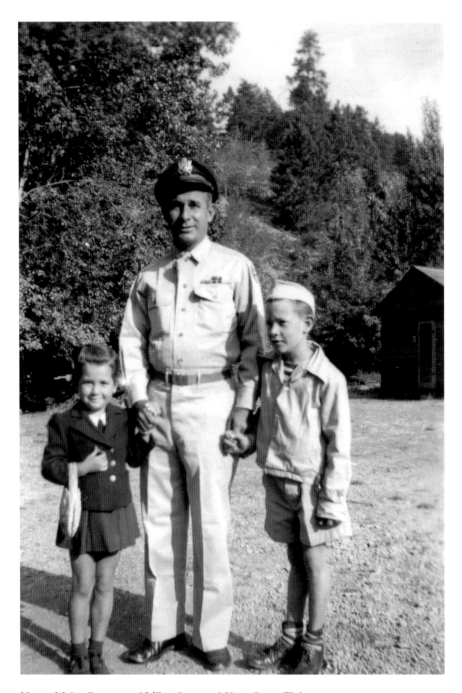

Nancy, Major Copass, and Mike. *Courtesy of Nancy Copass Tiederman.*

Michael started at Queen Anne High School in the eighth grade. There was no junior high in Seattle in those years. "That was a challenge because of bullying," he recalled. "But the first thing my dad did when he got back from the war was to buy two pair of boxing gloves, big ones for him and little ones for me, and taught me to box." One afternoon, his mother heard a big *splot* in the kitchen when his father gave him a bloody nose teaching him to defend himself. She ran down the basement stairs, demanding, "What are you doing to that boy?"

Her husband answered, "Teaching him to live with pain."

Dr. Copass's sister, Nancy, recalled these early accounts differently. She remembers her brother being casted for only about six months when he was six or seven years old. Furthermore, the only time she believes there was a fight was after she herself was hit in the head on purpose while playing kickball on a paved playground in the second grade. A boy threw a ball at her, knocking her out when her head struck the asphalt. Two days later, her fourth grade brother repeatedly pounded the kid in a very one-sided conflict. Aside from that, Michael Copass was a popular child, an Eagle Scout, consistently at the top of his high school class, a guard on the football team, and talented musically, but always a little shy and in awe of his father, and always in hope of measuring up to his standards, an age-old theme repeated about some boys and their fathers from the time of Philip and his son Alexander the Great to Theodore Roosevelt and his boy Teddy. The will to strive often requires an idealized competitor.

The character of the elder Mike Copass can be found spelled out in the letters that he wrote home during World War II, commentary on duty, honor, and dedication to others. In an undated letter (nonetheless noting the time as 1:00 a.m.) written from the U.S. Army Air Base in Sioux City, Iowa, Lieutenant Copass informs his younger sister about his decision to volunteer, saying, "I only hope that those who know and love me will understand how willingly and wholeheartedly I went to a duty I deeply felt, after my wife and I had carefully appraised all the sacrifice of separation, of business, and the like, which we as a family are making. When I think of these fine young boys undertaking training and combat risks a hundred times greater than mine, I could not leech off their blood and sleep again in peace." He complains that, for these same reasons, he could not spend the war "adjusting rents under the OPA."

All of these same values surfaced in the future physician's first experience as a paramedic at the age of ten. His father, in a letter to his own parents from his law office in 1949, wrote, "I thought you would be interested in seeing what a hero your grandson has become. I am sending you the front page of the *Post-Intelligencer* for May 14th, telling about how Mike witnessed a very bad accident involving three little boys, and jumped in the car and pulled on the hand brake. I did not understand why he had been gone so long when he returned and scolded him for being late. He simply told me that he had seen an accident and they had asked him to wait and tell what he knew."

In fact, young Mike knew a lot. "I'd gone to the library on my bike with my dog. I had permission to go. A woman in a dark blue Pontiac was turning right off McGraw onto 34th Street just as three boys entered the cross walk. She hit the first one, knocking him out of the way, and then ran over the other two. I saw the car was moving backwards over the boys, so I opened the driver's side door and pulled on the brake. Then I helped one of the firemen pull Jimmy Greenwood out from under the car, jumped on my bike, and furiously rode to the houses of the kids to tell their parents what had happened. I said that they had been taken to Swedish Hospital and that they should go there." But in fact, only two of them were taken by ambulance to Swedish. Jimmy Greenwood, age ten, died at the scene.

Copass's parents were dressed up and waiting to go out when he finally got home and told them he had been a witness to an accident and had given the police his name. But his parents thought he'd been goofing off instead, a mistake that sunk him "below the level of the earth." His father said, "I'll deal with you tomorrow." Then he told Carol, the babysitter, "If anybody comes, you call me."

Dr. Copass remembered years later, "Just after they left, the police arrived, but Carol didn't call. So I talked to the cops about legal stuff without a parent there. The question was, were the three boys in the crosswalk. They left, and a lawyer representing the driver knocked on the door. Then the prosecutor showed up."

Eventually, the case went to trial in Superior Court, and the lawyer father spent two days drilling his son on the questions he would be asked, including the fact that the boys had been in the crosswalk.

What Dr. Copass himself later internalized of this event was not his heroism, but the injustice of his father scolding him because he had come home late for dinner. "He had brown eyes that were so dark it seemed like you looked into a cave, and when he looked at you you knew he was looking right at you and they would burn a hole right through you. There was always a little smile, but he looked continually angry. In fact, in college he was called black Irish Mike," the son remembered of his father.

• • • •

In the summer of 1952, at the age of fourteen, Michael Copass hitchhiked to the Methow Valley in Eastern Washington for a job at the Sunny M dude ranch on land that has since become home to the Sun Mountain Lodge, a ski resort that looks over the valley above Patterson Lake. Most summers through medical school he lived on a big farm near Mesa, or on one of several other big farms in the eastern part of the state, working at outdoor jobs his father had helped him obtain through clients or friends.

Like many a fourteen-year-old boy, he was anxious to distance himself from that same father, although he certainly wanted to please him and to be found manly. At Queen Anne High, "if a friend needed someone to finish the fight or take care of the wounded on the ground it was my job; I was the closer. There is a certain degree of baloney that goes on in high school. As my son is teaching my grandsons, we don't bully, push, or shove people who are smaller than we are, defenseless, or female. That lesson hung on to me for the rest of my life."

Indeed, his father was a heroic figure for a variety of reasons, but the lesson that dominated family life in the Copass household during the McCarthy era came from the Seattle HUAC hearings. Following the war, the senior Copass had had a hard time reigniting his law practice until he partnered with his colleague and friend Jack McWalter. A Scot born in Glasgow, McWalter was a marine law specialist, and the firm of Copass and McWalter had been doing well. In 1952, after years of pipe smoking, McWalter suddenly died in bed, and the legal business again slowed for the senior Copass. Eventually, Governor Art Langley appointed him to be a judge in the King County Superior Court. From there, he went on to become the president of the King County Bar Association just as the communist scare accelerated. When a Seattle citizen named Stanley Henrickson was hauled before the committee, no one rushed to defend him. In a June 1954 article, the *Seattle Times* reported that former judge Mike Copass had volunteered to represent Henrickson, stating that every person "has an absolute right to advice of council where life and liberty are concerned, irrespective of the rights of the matter." For this acceptance of his duty, hate phone calls came in and rocks were several times thrown through the windows of the family home. Young Mike and Nancy were instructed not to answer the telephone and to keep away from the windows.

Of his graduation as the valedictorian of his class at Queen High School and one of the commencement speakers, Copass later said, "I made it though high school and decided I don't want to go to the 13th grade. I thought that's what UW was, and that was a wrong assumption on my part." Eventually, somebody from Yale interviewed him, an event he found frightening. No teacher or counselor had told him where he should go to school or what he should study after he graduated in 1956, so he decided to join the army.

But he didn't. The way he remembers it, "My good friend Bill Warren, whose dad ran KOMO, said he was going to Stanford and I thought that was a pretty good deal. So I applied to the Leland Stanford, Jr. University, not thinking that I would get in. But I got in without any trouble, and then in the summer of 1956 I hitchhiked from the farm where I

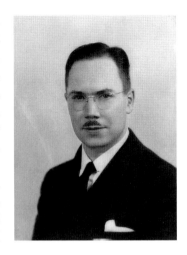

Jack McWalter in law school, about age thirty. *Courtesy of Bryce McWalter.*

worked near the Tri Cities, to Pasco, to John Day, Oregon, to Sacramento, to Palo Alto." He carried all his possessions in his dad's wartime air force "B-4" bag and recalled riding some distance with a minister so drunk he sang, "Hallelujah, we are on our way" for the entire trip.

"It must have worked, because we missed hitting anything."

Mike's sister, Nancy, claims that Stanford was greatly valued in the family, and to her it was predictable that both she and her brother would attend college there, as both of them did.

At Stanford, Mike majored in biology and chemistry and studied history. When his sister arrived two years later, she dated one of his fraternity brothers, who thought it was ridiculous how much she admired her brother, who had hung a copy of the Kipling poem "IF" above his desk. The final stanza seems to have helped inform his life.

If you can talk with crowds and keep your virtue,
Or walk with Kings—nor lose the common touch,
If neither foes nor loving friends can hurt you,
If all men count with you, but none too much;
If you can fill the unforgiving minute
With sixty seconds' worth of distance run,
Yours is the Earth and everything that's in it,
And—which is more—you'll be a Man, my son!

But even more important than Rudyard Kipling, it was at Stanford that Mike met Lucy Ames, a young woman from Fairfax County, Virginia. "I was interested in International Relations and learned Russian in the wake of Sputnik, which had captured the country. I had the choice of an East Coast school, a Midwest school, or Stanford. My dad, who had a good sense of humor, said, 'Well, it comes down to what kind of a man you want to marry.' Because I had been enchanted as a teenager with Owen Wister (I fell in love with the cowboy in his novel *The Virginian*, and his novels about Winthrop, Washington), so I said to my dad only somewhat facetiously, 'Well, I want to marry a cowboy'. He replied, 'Go west, young woman, go west.' Turned out when I met Mike on a blind date he was wearing his jeans and cowboy boots recounting his rodeo experiences in Winthrop."

When asked how long it took him to know this was the person he wanted to marry, Copass answered, "An hour and a half." They met in the fall of 1958, her freshman year, when he was a junior.

. . . .

Mike entered medical school at Northwestern University straight from college. Lucy worked for the Peace Corps as a volunteer before she graduated and then joined the Peace Corps and worked for Sargent Shriver in Washington, D.C. Mike commuted to Palo Alto and later to D.C. every available weekend to see her.

At Northwestern, he developed an interest in general surgery because he considered it an active kind of work. He went to work in the lab of John Bergan, a vascular surgeon who did the first kidney transplant in Chicago. Mike's job was to make a small bowel obstruction, so he mastered superior mesenteric artery occlusion and knew more about it than his supervisors. But then he had to keep the specimen alive, so he also became an intensivist for dogs twelve hours a day.

To help pay the bills, he worked in the clinical lab at Wesley Memorial Hospital nights and weekends. These were valuable jobs handed down from med student to med student. Mike and a roommate shared that same lab job but worked opposite shifts, so while they had a single-bed apartment, they were never there at the same time and got by paying only one rent.

He home-delivered babies through the Chicago Maternity Center on an obstetrics rotation and made some money nights and weekends checking patients' charts at the Teamsters Clinic. "One night an angry teamster decided I was a pain in the ass because I made him show me all his ID and then told him it was a buck and a half to see the doctor, who was an Ob-Gyn resident. So he grabbed the cash register with a gigantic hand and threw it at me. That was a crazy place to be at night."

The summer before Lucy and Mike married, he lived with Bill and Ruth Nagel, an aunt and uncle of Nancy's husband. Ruth was part Choctaw Indian, and Bill was a full-blooded Irishman who knew most of the cops in Chicago. After the hurled cash register episode, Uncle Bill got his nephew a slightly safer job with a trucking company helping to move valuables out of strong boxes, which were periodically inspected by the IRS and valued for tax purposes. More importantly, Bill Nagel used his connections to the trucking firm to get Mike on moving vans bound for Washington, D.C., where Lucy was working for the Peace Corps.

At the 1962 Seattle World's Fair, Mike and Lucy got engaged. At first, Mike's father opposed the union. Although he adored Lucy, he felt that his son shouldn't marry just then because he was unable to support a wife. Mike senior felt so strongly that he flew to Chicago to try to convince them they couldn't afford to marry.

"Show me the budget, Mike," he told me. "I let him know I wouldn't have too many more chances and I'd better take this one. He thought I should finish training first, mostly because he worried about money from his own experience."

They got married anyway, in January 1963, and then Mike drove to Washington to move Lucy to Chicago with him for his last year at Northwestern.

They left the Beltway headed west and ran out of gas on the Ohio Turnpike when the car's sediment bowl (a primitive gas line filter) froze. "We were picked off the highway by a guy driving a Consolidated Freightways set of doubles who saw we were distressed, looking like whipped puppies, and took us to the next station." Then the gas station attendant drove back to the car, took off the sediment bowl and warmed it in his hands enough to get the gas flowing. He returned with the car to the station, and the newlyweds went on to Chicago in the middle of a blizzard. Driving up the Dan Ryan on two inches of ice and snow Lucy broke down and cried. Mike thought, perhaps in the voice of his father, "I've brought this wonderful girl into a mess."

They found an unfurnished apartment for $39.00 a month on the now gentrified Wrightwood Avenue just off Clarke Street. They walked to a furniture store off Lake Shore Drive and for $41.50 bought a round pine table and chairs that came from the Board Room of the First National Bank of Chicago—which they still have.

The newlyweds had no idea what they were going to do when he graduated in the coming June 1964.

Though he had applied to several surgical programs, a little girl in the hospital exposed Mike to the measles just when the interviews were about to begin. Because he was an adult, he was very sick, and having no money, he could not have visited the programs he'd applied to even had he been well. By that time, the intern match had begun, but because he hadn't interviewed anywhere, he didn't match. With some scurrying around, he was invited to stay at Wesley Memorial for his intern year. This event he viewed as a major failure. He was embarrassed to have to tell his father about it.

. . . .

He was immediately drafted into the army when he finished the internship in 1965 and was sent to Fort Sam Houston for basic training. From there, the army assigned him to the 11th Air Assault Group, stationed at Fort Sill, Oklahoma. But he never made it to Oklahoma because a soldier who was supposed to go to Europe with a different outfit refused to give them a required extra third year of service for such a good post. So that soldier went to the 11th Air Assault in Mike's place, then to Vietnam, and Mike went to Europe. He felt so guilty about getting the safer assignment he wanted to go back to Fort Sill. "Lucy had a short fuse, and it was lit. She attacked me," he remembered. The way his wife tells it, "I was so relieved when he said he didn't have to go. And then when he said he was going to volunteer, meaning Vietnam, even though I'm a non-violent person, I slapped him."

Instead of Vietnam, they went to Frankfurt, Germany. As a battalion surgeon to the headquarters of the 5th Corps, he spent months "waiting in the Fulda Gap east of Frankfurt for the Russians to invest themselves on the German plain."

His duties were to take care of the health and welfare of 1,200 soldiers, and part of the way he achieved that was to hold sick call every morning from nine o'clock to noon. This was an effort to sort out who was really ill from those who were sick of the work. Fortunately, he had with him Harry Paxton, a very good NCO who had been at his job for a long time and understood the army. Paxton was the author of the great two-word speech "Fuckin' fucker, you fuckin' fucker…" He ran the dispensary and, when riled, often asked, "Should I give you the two-word speech?" Everybody trembled. "Harry Paxton was a hard man to fool. He was the best nonphysician at diagnosis that I've ever seen in my life. And he could really understand bullshit."

Mike's tour would have been up in 1967, but his dad had just died (a malignant brain tumor first misdiagnosed as several small strokes) and he and Lucy had decided to have a baby, so he signed on for a third year. Their daughter Clo, named for her aunt, was born in that year, and Mike was then reassigned to Berchtesgaden, where he was the commander of the 13th Medical Detachment until discharged in 1968.

In Berchtesgaden, and Germany in general, they had designed excellent helicopter rescue operations with aircraft units assigned to the hospitals. They flew Sikorsky Choctaws, with the engines mounted in front of the aircraft. "We would move really sick people from Berchtesgaden to Munich. One night in blinding Bavarian rain a soldier who had been on a religious retreat pondering the meaning of life and God had a GI bleed because the pondering was more than he could take. So we flew him with a very low hematocrit to Munich. The only fluids I had were saline and albumen. All of a sudden there is a burning on the back of my neck, and the grizzled old crew chief standing behind me says 'Aw, don't worry, doc, it's just the hydraulic fluid for the rotor actuators. I got a fix for it right here.' He reached in a back pocket and out comes a greasy old rag that he wrapped around the leaking hydraulic line. Out of another pocket came a vice grip that he snapped on the rag. 'We'll stay in the air now,' he said when the leak stopped."

Copass claimed, "The army was an interesting time for me because I like order. I liked the fact that there were inspections we had to get ready for and we had to figure out how to get around them. To prove that all our weapons were in good shape, we sent them off to the armory just before inspection. Eleven machine guns and AR-15, all in the armory being cared for by the armorer." They did faithfully keep all the injection records, however, and everyone was up to date on the immunizations.

"One of the things I did in Berchtesgaden was to take care of nineteen intelligence units, guys who were really busy snatching Russian soldiers and military people out of Czechoslovakia. It was kind of like Guantanamo. They didn't water board then, they just talked to them all day long. They were funny guys too. The one in charge was an ex-sergeant in the Polish army and was not a friend of anything Russian. There were a couple of big, African American guys from Texas who had been to the Army Language School in Monterey, California, who could speak Russian, Lucy said, without a southern accent."

When the army career ended in 1968, there wasn't much waiting for him at home because he hadn't really been in any program, much less embarked on the study of any specific medical specialty when he had departed.

He had hoped to rejoin the medicine residency at Northwestern. An attending physician there had written to him in the army telling him to return because they had a slot for him. But on the day of the proposed start of the residency, the faculty members he met told him he had to interview again. He did. They were talking about phenformin lactic acidosis at noon rounds: "I knew as much about that as I did nuclear theory. I knew a lot about an AR-15, and how to change the track and rebuild the engine on an armored personnel carrier, how to set up a machine gun and shoot it, how to guarantee that my dispensary was fortified, and where to put the x-ray machine." He despaired of finding a residency.

"After I flunked phenformin lactic acidosis, I was sent to talk to the chair, who asked me what I wanted to do, and I said I wasn't sure. Then he asked me what I read, and I told him *Munich Medical Week*, *The New England Journal*, and *The Berlin Medical Week*. We also have *Izvestia* around the house because Lucy is interested in Russian." The professor and chairman of the Department of Medicine at Northwestern University School of Medicine then looked over the top of his glasses and asked the applicant, "Would you be interested in what I read?" Dr. Copass later recalled, "I was maybe a little snippy when I said to him 'if you read more than *Time* I'd be really surprised.' Not the right answer."

Knowing full well that he was not going to stay in Chicago, he took the redeye to Seattle. Lucy and Clo were staying in Oklahoma with Nancy. This was another major disappointment to the young Dr. Copass, who did not want to return to Seattle and live, he believed, in the giant shadow of his father's reputation.

"First thing I did was stop at Harborview to see Dr. Harold Laws, who then was the hospital director." Interestingly, Mike's father had been a close friend of Dr. Laws's. "I can't give you a job but go out the university and talk to the Chair of Medicine, Dr. Petersdorf," he told me. "I took the bus to the U and saw the Dorf and asked for a job as an internist. He said there are no openings. Just as I got up to leave, he said the neurologists need some help, so I went and found Phil Swanson, the chairman. He was interesting. He found me sitting reading *Science*, and he pulled a neurology journal off the shelf and said, 'Here, this will be more useful to you.' He threw it at me, and then offered me a job, so I suddenly became a neurology resident. I was a sandbag; they needed to fill up the space in the dike."

His first rotation was as a second-year resident at what was then the Children's Orthopedic Hospital, in the days on-call residents stayed in the hospital for twenty-four hours straight. His call room assignment was in the female residents' call room. After listening to the commotion all night and being kept out of the bathroom in the morning while several women showered, dressed, and put on makeup, he decided he didn't want to be there. So he began to set the alarm clock to ring early so he could shower first and shave before the women woke up. They weren't happy about the situation either and were relieved to lose their guest.

"I loved the COH rotation. I had an interesting experience treating *status epilepticus*. A kid with Sturge Weber had a terrible seizure disorder, was convulsing and wouldn't stop. A peds resident asked me what to do, and I said we'd used paraldehyde at Wesley. He said we don't use that here and suggested phenobarbital. 'OK, give me a laryngoscope, an endotracheal tube, and put them right there with five-hundred mg of phenobarb.' So I pushed it in, the fits stopped and, needless to say, so did his breathing. So I flipped him sideways with his head hanging off the side of the bed and intubated him before they could spit. After that, the peds residents and I got along great. On the day they all met for professors' rounds, the chief came with a big folder filled with articles from *Redbook*, *Reader's Digest*, etc. He said, 'This is your reading for the month. If you know these you'll know what people are doing and thinking.' I thought that was brilliant."

Dr. Mike Copass was a University of Washington neurology resident from 1969 to 1972. Most people thought he often behaved more like a surgeon than an internist. Indeed, agreed his sister, at Northwestern he did want to be a surgeon but feared he wouldn't be able to stand at the operating table on the knee he injured playing as an undersized 150-pound guard on the Queen Anne High School football team. That never hindered his standing all day in the emergency room.

PORTABLE 55

B y the time Copass finished his neurology training, Medic One was in operation, though not securely funded. The $28,000 first Mobile Intensive Coronary Care Unit, Moby Pig, went on the streets in March 1970, and by then, Len Cobb and colleagues had trained nineteen firefighters in how to manage cardiac emergencies. They were already saving crucial time by beginning treatment at the scene, bypassing the ER, and admitting patients directly to a still very basic intensive care unit.

In 1969, HMC Chief of Medicine Bob Conn had started the first Coronary Care Unit at Harborview.[20] The hospital rebuilt an eight-bed ward on Four Center into its first ICU. Chief Resident Len Hudson's office adjoined the space, which had a window opening into the unit, a ward that Conn had asked him to manage. There was no real faculty interest because at the time no one yet knew much about how to provide care in a specialized coronary unit, so Dr. Hudson, the junior residents, and the nurses managed patients at the same time they were learning what worked best. Medic One brought them a regular delivery of cardiac patients.

In a May 1970 article in the *Seattle P-I*, Charles Russell wrote, "Yesterday three such patients were recovering in Seattle hospitals. One, a 44-year old man restored to life after a heart attack Wednesday, wanted to play cards with his rescuers."[21] Even so, by late in 1970, the grant that was supposed to pay the bills for two and a half years was already running dry.

In the first six months of operation, paramedics had responded to 630 calls and treated 83 patients in ventricular fibrillation, a life-threatening

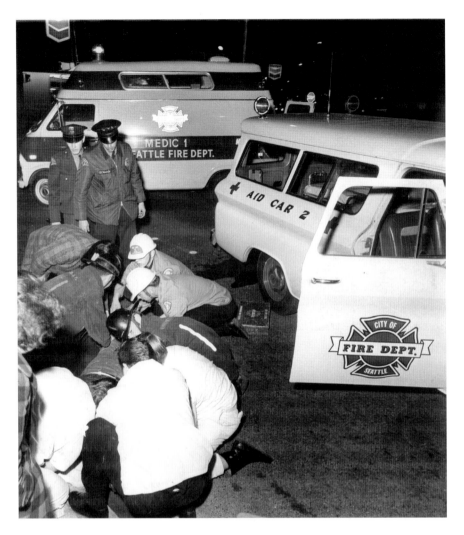

Aid car and EMTs at work, early 1970s. *Courtesy of Seattle Fire Department.*

condition. Both of the major Seattle daily papers began to howl for a more durable method of funding the Seattle Medic One program. In a commentary titled "A Case of Mickey Mouse Municipal Management" aired on February 1, 1971, KVI news commentator Bob Roberts said he was happy to be reassured that "Medic One will not be allowed to go out of service for lack of funds."[22] Less optimistically, he added, "that very assurance reinforces the cussed notion we've got that the present city administration cannot attend to anything beyond routine matters of

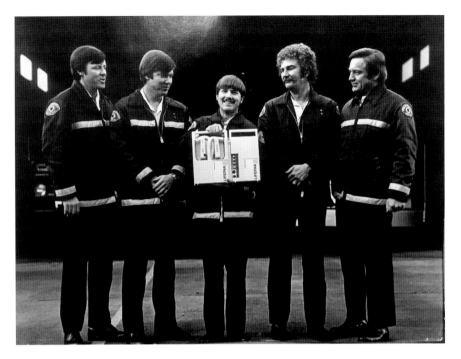

Paramedics display Physio Control LifePak 5 defibrillator, late 1970s. (*Left to right*)
Paramedics Rick Smith, Roy Waugh, Chuck Kahler, Zane Wyll, A.D. Vickery. *Courtesy of Medic One.*

public business without first dancing a chorus of 'Waltz Me Around Again, Willie,' with the public."

While the mayor and the city council waltzed around the budget constraints, Gordon Vickery stepped a ballroom dance lunge into action, and he was graceful at it. In January 1971, he sent a memo to the fire department staff describing how to collect donations for Medic One, announcing a two-week public subscription drive. In February of that year, Vickery assembled a board headed by Henry Broderick, president of the board of Henry Broderick Inc; Paul Friedlander, president of Friedlander & Sons; Lloyd Coony, president of KIRO; and Hunter Simpson, president of Physio-Control, and began to organize the fundraising. They appealed for money through the newspapers, radio, and TV stations, and even with signs along the highways. Firefighters shook tin cups out on the streets, and businesses all over town contributed to the drive to save Medic One. The Ballard VFW came up with $1,000. The Seattle Restaurant Association, Rainier Brewery, Safeco Insurance, Teamsters Local 117, automobile dealerships, cocktail

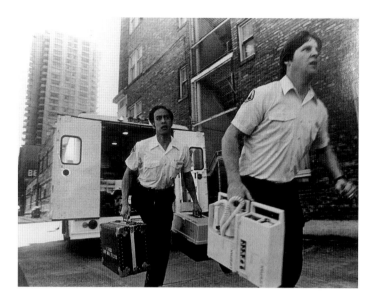

Early paramedics Ed Edwards (*front*) and Randy Foy in promotional ad for Physio Control, late 1970s. *Courtesy of Seattle Fire Department.*

lounges, and at least one barbershop also donated. By the first of March, they had raised about half of their goal amount, so Vickery turned up the heat with more announcements.

The campaign was starting to make elected public officials look bad, and they knew it. In reply, King County executive John Spellman convened a meeting of city and county agencies in an effort to expand the Medic One program to the county and to find more money. They didn't get very far.[23]

The young mayor, Wes Uhlman, whom the Seattle establishment sometimes referred to as the kid from the U, had to learn quickly about pre-hospital care. "It was pitched," he said years later, "as something that would not be a long term cost for the city, and even in the short term not much money."[24] But the Boeing company was nearly going broke during the first eight months he was mayor, and on April 16, 1971, two real estate agents put up the famous sign near Sea-Tac International Airport: "Will the Last Person Leaving Seattle—Turn Out the Lights."

Uhlman found that the biggest opposition to Medic One came from the private operators, mainly Shepard Ambulance. Although they had had patient transport all to themselves for years, ambulances were slower and more expensive than Medic One and not really operated by qualified emergency responders with current training in advanced life support. A Shepard representative came to his office very early on and told Mayor Uhlman, "This will put us out of business." The company could not compete and eventually did go out of business, inasmuch as that it was ultimately sold to AMR in 1995.

There was no opposition from the City of Seattle other than the competing budget forces. So far as the mayor was concerned, "It was a Vickery program. Years before when I was actively practicing law, I'd been a little bit involved with the private ambulance companies so I knew the turf." In fact, for a while before he was elected mayor, Uhlman had represented Shepard legal interests. Within a year, the city bureaucracy was in full support of Medic One, a short time by bureaucratic standards. "But the union didn't necessarily like the idea," Uhlman later said. "In those days, they considered themselves to be firemen. Then they got smart and saw that it meant more jobs and more pay."

Thirty-seven years after he left office as mayor, Uhlman said, "Medic One worked in Seattle because people cooperated and Vickery understood the concept and could execute. I had confidence in him. I give him 85 percent of the credit."

When the fire department itself came up with the money it had pledged to raise in 1971, Chief Vickery wrote to the staunch, though seldom conventional, Medic One supporter Bob Hardwick, a disc jockey at KVI radio, who answered, thanking him by declaring, "Chief, I'd set myself on fire for you!" Vickery ended his reply by writing, "This letter is to let you know we are happy to accept your offer. If you'll just let me know the time and place, we'll be pleased to notify the press."[25] The chief knew how to use the press. By the end of the month, the campaign to save Medic One had raised a total of $146,421.

Hoping to maximize the use of these dollars for Medic One only, and not to allow the total to be diluted by passing through the UW School of Medicine, which extracts various taxes for its own operations, Cobb first deposited the money raised with the Beacon Hill Research Foundation.[26] A board managed this money, used solely to fund the fire department's emergency services. In 1974, the Medic One Foundation took over the responsibility of both fundraising and expanding the program, which is currently financed by local property tax levies voted on by the public every six years, plus those contributions made by private and business donations.

It is certainly true that because of the economic slowdown both city and county governments had budget constraints in 1971, so while the public agitated to expand the Medic One program, there was little reply and not much happened. On June 14, the *Seattle Times* Editorial Board wrote, "County dallies on Medic One," and called King County's reluctance to expand on the early successes "deplorable."

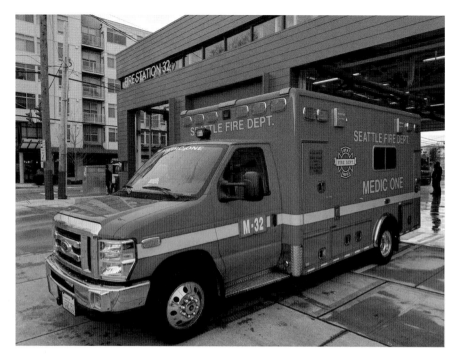

Medic One rig in West Seattle, 1970–80s. *Courtesy of Seattle Fire Department.*

By then, 911 had become the number to call in case of emergency all over the country, making response times much faster. KIRO televised an editorial about an employee at its station who had collapsed on the job. "It was exactly two minutes from the time someone dialed 911 until the first aid car was on the scene. Less than two minutes later, Medic One, with its lifesaving equipment, was also here." Things began to move.

The underpowered and bouncy Moby Pig lasted just a year, and then a Ballard body shop replaced it with a dedicated, well-designed Ford truck rebuilt into an emergency rig.

In the fall of 1971, Dr. Cobb and Chief Vickery announced the "Medic Two" program. A $100,000 grant from Seattle Rotary (Chief Vickery was a member) and another $9,000 from the Washington State Heart Association (to which Cobb belonged) aimed to fund CPR training for willing citizens. On October 21, the *Seattle P-I* reported that "the program will be open to all Seattle residents, including older children, and will be taught by Medic One personnel."

In 1973, 18,000 Seattle citizens learned CPR from Seattle medics. Over the next two years, that number reached Vickery and Cobb's goal of teaching

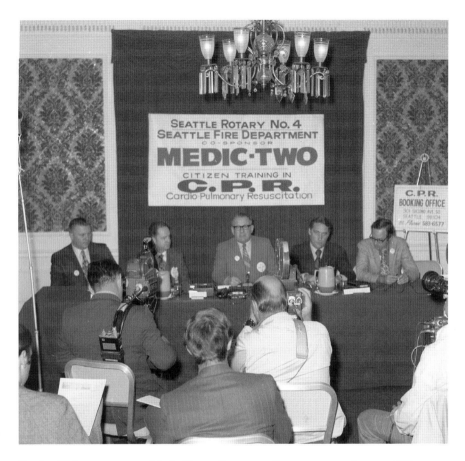

Gordon Vickery announces Medic Two at Downtown Rotary press conference, 1971. *Courtesy of Medic One Foundation, Jennifer Blackwood.*

100,000 ordinary people how to save the life of someone who had collapsed, wasn't breathing, or was pulseless.[27]

From its inception until 1972, paramedics could only ride Medic One and treat patients if a doctor was on the rig with them. During the day, hospital medicine residents provided this service (because they were told to and needed the experience), and at night internal medicine and cardiology attendings made the runs (because they wanted to). Personnel on the Medic One rigs required supervision because various medical interests had opposed the idea that high school graduates—the educational level of most of the firefighters who became paramedics then—could be trained to do what physicians had gone to college and four years of medical school to learn. When he was asked about this obstruction much later, Pat Fleet, a dedicated, gravel-voiced, no-nonsense Harborview internal medicine attending in those years, surprised the questioner by saying, "Of course they can. Just think about looking around at your med school classmates."[28]

In 1972, the law finally changed and allowed paramedics independent standing to treat patients, thereby eliminating the need for the direct physician supervision on the rigs. Doctors would always have medical control remotely from Harborview or, depending on the fire district, other hospitals. The persisting problem was an absence of direct faculty supervision over what was morphing from an emergency room into the Harborview Emergency Department because, like all big county hospitals of the era, residents ran the ER. While there might have been attendings to help guide treatment during business hours, the residents were there all night on their own. By late in 1973, when Copass became the director of emergency services at Harborview, a whole new way of managing the growing department began to take form.

• • • •

One thing that didn't change was Leonard Cobb's commitment to gathering data. By 1973, he had collected the first three years of experience examining Medic One pre-hospital care. He and coauthor Al "Crazy Al" Alvarez, so named because despite his known bleeding disorder he still loved to race cars and motorcycles, published their findings in 1974.[29]

During the first three years in operating a comprehensive system for the management of out-of-hospital medical emergencies, 146 patients were resuscitated from ventricular fibrillation, hospitalized, and discharged home. The diagnosis of acute transmural myocardial infarction associated with the episode of ventricular fibrillation was confirmed in only 17 percent of the patients.

It is concluded that: 1) out-of-hospital ventricular fibrillation is common and treatable; 2) the phenomenon of sudden cardiac death should not be equated with acute myocardial infarction; 3) patients resuscitated from ventricular fibrillation without associated acute myocardial infarction are prone to sudden death—most likely from ventricular fibrillation.

In 1975, they reported a total of two hundred thirty-four patients with ventricular fibrillation treated in the field, resuscitated, hospitalized, and discharged to home since Medic One hit the streets, or about 50 patients saved per year.[30]

Now it was Frank Pantridge in Ireland who read the journals and became excited about work being done in America that seemed to substantiate his ideas concerning pre-hospital care. In the early 1970s, he visited Seattle and other American cities eager to validate the concept he called "pre-hospital mobile coronary care" with data. In fact, he found his work was received more warmly in this country than in Ireland or the UK.

Professor Jennifer Adgey, who was an early Pantridge colleague, has held the position of consultant cardiologist at the Royal Victoria Hospital since 1971.[31] She remembered that

> *he visited Dr. Bill Grace in New York, Dr. Lewis in Columbus, Dr. Dick Crampton in Charlottesville, and Dr. Stanley Sarnoff in Washington, D.C. He recognized that the majority of deaths from coronary artery disease occurred outside the hospital due to cardiac arrest and hoped that the U.S. evidence would support his ideas. Most cardiologists worldwide ignored this data and put many obstacles in the way of doctors attempting to address the problem by failing mainly to support initial efforts such as those occurring in our group. I think it is fair to say that very few cardiologists in the UK at that time supported out of hospital coronary care. In fact there were several publications in or around 1966 indicating that there was no point in treating patients with myocardial infarction outside the hospital as the mortality was the same as those first treated inside hospital. Pantridge also felt that the Americans understood his approach much better. Indeed it took approximately ten years for cardiologists in the UK to grudgingly accept that out of hospital coronary care was beneficial. This was long after the time paramedic units had been established in the U.S. to manage cardiac patients outside the hospital.*

Though a grateful guest in Seattle, Pantridge could be difficult for people who disagreed with him, and he alienated a number of them. He was direct about his opinions, even confrontational, and occasionally called people stupid and arrogant even though he didn't really have a lot of good data of his own. What he did have in Belfast were defibrillators designed for hospital use that had "to be plugged into the mains," meaning into a 230 wall socket. So in the winter of 1965, Pantridge, his senior house officer John Geddes, and a technician converted one of these 150-pound hospital machines to operate powered by two twelve-volt DC car batteries through a static invertor and were soon hauling around a modified defibrillator in an ancient ambulance manned by Geddes. It was "a huge sucker," said Dr. Cobb, "so they did defibrillate some people, though his principle contention was that you could improve the outcomes of people with acute MI by earlier intervention:

Lidocaine, morphine, and shocking them. He wasn't interested in trauma. He liked it that we were keeping records on pre-hospital emergency care and publishing complete data."

Soon thereafter, the Irish professor invited Cobb to a meeting of the Royal College of Physicians (Cardiology) in Belfast. It was still in the days of the Troubles in Northern Ireland, and not that long after the August riots of 1969. The Royal Victoria Hospital campus is vast and bordered on one side by Falls Road, a main thoroughfare that had been the scene of clashes between Catholics and Protestants. In fact, the Sinn Fein office was located on Falls Road. Because he had stayed with them in Seattle, Pantridge had the gift of an Irish linen tablecloth made for Cobb and his wife, Else, at a small local shop down Falls Road from the hospital. Due to the Troubles, which at the time could be punctuated by explosions, shootings, and beatings, he didn't want Cobb to go get the linen alone, so he sent his secretary with him to pick it up. At least, he reasoned, she would know what was unsafe. On their way, an armored car came by with guns drawn looking for snipers. The secretary sped up. After a few more blocks, they reached the shop, knocked, waited long enough for the door to open a crack, grabbed the linen, and fled. Though alarmed, they made it back to the hospital unmolested.

· · · ·

At about the same time during his first year as director of the ED at Harborview, Dr. Copass spent his time organizing the new world of emergency care. Now they were managing not only cardiac events but also trauma of every sort. Medicine and surgery residents on rotation in the ED became responsible for supervising the care of the patient from the moment they were picked up by the paramedics until they were admitted into the hospital. A second-year medicine resident became the Medic One doc, who managed the cardiac events, and a second-year surgery resident was the trauma doc and managed everything else. By this time, paramedics were credentialed by the change in the law and therefore recognized by the state. In 1975, a brand-new state-of-the-art ED opened at Harborview on the north end of the building, and what had been the old ER vanished, both physically and from memory.

Emergency vehicles now drove in under cover to the double doors entering straight into a registration desk, where nurses triaged very sick patients with acute problems to either medicine or surgery. Those less ill waited in rooms down the hall to the right just past the decontamination room used for cleaning up the lice-infected. Acute surgical patients went straight ahead into one of the four trauma bays or down a parallel long hall to the dedicated Emergency Department x-ray suite for plain films. Two acute medicine beds were beyond the trauma bays and beyond that a room where they put the pus (that is, septic or otherwise so infected patients that they were a hazard to others). The "fish bowl," the glassed-in room just past triage separating it from the trauma bays, became the nerve center under the command of Dr. Copass, and he didn't miss much even before he became known as "Portable 55."

In an age long before cellphones, Portable 55 appeared because Al Alvarez, a cardiology fellow at the time, was in on the original Medic One training faculty and wanted to have instant communication between the ED and the medics. The radiophones they all carried to begin with were enormous in comparison to modern devices, but thanks to upgrades at the Fire Department Alarm Center, they were a huge improvement over the old-fashioned fire alarm boxes, which by then had been removed. Alvarez became Portable 33, and Dwayne Beatz, who had been a trauma fellow in Dallas with Tom Shires, the recently recruited and controversial new chairman of the Department of Surgery at UW, was the first dedicated ED surgeon known as Portable 44. That designation now belongs to the Seattle Fire Department Medical Services Officer (MSO) on duty daily to manage Medic One in Seattle.

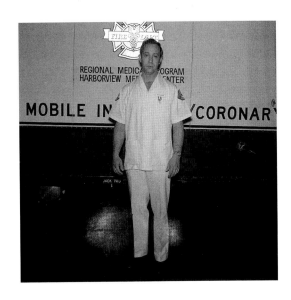

Barry Newcomb, one of the first paramedics, and Moby Pig. *Courtesy of SD Vickery.*

At that time, and for the next thirty-five years, Mike Copass read every patient chart and all the logs the paramedics kept of their runs for appropriateness, completeness, accuracy, and anything else he might want to argue about over what had happened to that patient. "What I wanted to know was the chief complaint and did we work up everything completely. If we didn't, I marked the chart. And if we took too long, or goofed off, I marked the chart. I looked at the time in and out." Everyone who worked in the ED, or rotated through it, remembers with dread finding, printed in orange wax x-ray film–marking crayon on top of a chart, the Copass note "SEE ME," or even worse, "WTF." This was long before texting. SEE ME meant he thought you'd missed something, were incomplete, took too long, ordered the wrong tests, or otherwise didn't measure up to his standard and required education. WTF meant you were in for it. This process began at six o'clock in the morning, and he was often still there late at night. At the same time, he attended in neurology three months a year, alternating with Mark Sumi, Colie Carlson, and later Will Longstreth, now the longtime chief of neurology at HMC. He ran Medic One. He also held his own clinic once a week, an undertaking dedicated not only to diseases of the nervous system but really open to any patient who wanted to see him for any reason. Dr. Copass's first rule was, "If someone asks for help, you give him help."

Two other notations might appear on the Medic One logs and ED charts.[32] By this time, the paramedics were devoted to Mike Copass and he to them. He also knew and was known by most of the Seattle cops. His day always began having coffee with the two Medic One Medical Services Officers, one beginning a twenty-four-hour shift and the other going home. When dispatched to pick up someone the medics discovered were colleagues or acquaintances of the ED director, "FOC" appeared on the top of the record—Friend of Copass. The night Len Hudson, professor of medicine and longtime beloved chief of pulmonology at Harborview, thought he might be having an MI and called Medic One, a couple of the paramedics who arrived stared at him curiously. Once they finally recognized him, they took him straight to the hospital, not as Dr. Hudson, but as "FOC." In those same years, Kathy Fair was Hudson's patient-care coordinator, a position they invented together. Kathy was enormously efficient and organized, so she could keep track of patients as they moved from the ED throughout the system and follow up with them after discharge. If Copass was worried about a patient disappearing or at risk of being unable to manage follow-up, he wrote "FAIR" on the ED chart so Kathy could track the person, prompting more than one medicine resident to wonder aloud, "What does it take to get a 'good' around here?" Kathy Fair later also worked for Medic One.

Robert Jetland was the chief executive officer at Harborview then, and he was enthusiastic about Medic One, knowing it would bring patients and offer them a far greater chance at survival. "The Jet" was also on the board of the Medic One Foundation, as were Len Cobb, Dean of the Medical School Robert Van Citters, and Jack Richards, who had replaced Gordon Vickery as the fire chief when Vickery became the director of Seattle City Light. Harold Laws was still the medical director at Harborview. They all gave Medic One enthusiastic support.

So did *60 Minutes*, when Morley Safer told the nation in 1974, "If you're going to have a heart attack, have it in Seattle." The story showed Safer riding in the back of one of the Medic One rigs explaining to his viewers that you were more likely to survive a heart attack in Seattle than anywhere else in the country. At the time, that also meant anywhere in the world.

While the rest of the country and the world were busy admiring the Medic One system, in Seattle, the fire department budget remained a problem. Again Mayor Uhlman wound up in the middle of a controversy: his 1974 proposal to the city council that the Budget Office study whether "Expensive and highly trained Medic One fire fighters should be replaced by civilian paramedics."[33] This was an unpopular suggestion made worse by speculation that Uhlman, an attorney for the Shepard Ambulance Company before becoming mayor, might have had conflicted motivations. Not too surprisingly, the firefighters certainly believed that he did. While no evidence supported the rumor, a lot of people thought about it. On October 13, 1974, *Seattle Times* editorialist Herb Robinson wrote, "Uhlman's tinkering with Medic One is a political Enigma."[34] Public outcry and editorials in both papers soon caused the mayor to back down. On October 18, 1974, the *Seattle Post-Intelligencer* quoted Uhlman's letter to Councilman Tim Hill, chair of the budget committee, which stated, "The response to even the suggestion of examining our Medic One program has been so strong that I am convinced our citizens do not want any changes in the program for any reason."[35]

Assured of more secure financing, Cobb, Floyd Short, Al Alvarez, and Robert Miller started improving the early EMT training classes. "Alvarez took an active interest in being the boss. He liked the idea of driving a fire engine," Dr. Cobb remembered. The goal of the training was to teach them to do what a well-trained doctor would do if he were there: intubate, put

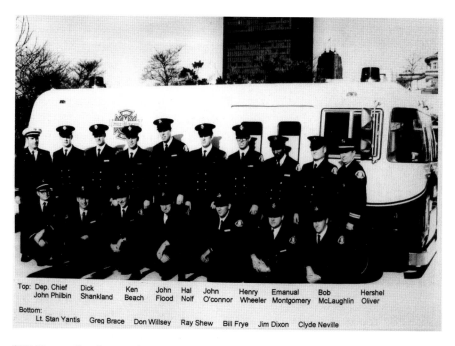

Top: Dep. Chief Dick Ken John Hal John Henry Emanual Bob Hershel
John Philbin Shankland Beach Flood Nolf O'connor Wheeler Montgomery McLaughlin Oliver
Bottom:
Lt. Stan Yantis Greg Brace Don Willsey Ray Shew Bill Frye Jim Dixon Clyde Neville

SFD Paramedics class number one and Moby Pig, 1970. *Courtesy of Seattle Fire Department.*

in central lines, give IV fluids to resuscitate, pass a nasogastric tube, get a twelve-lead EKG, start CPR. Paramedics soon learned to evaluate chest and abdominal trauma and then began to reduce open fractures, something that initially irritated the community orthopedists who were convinced only they should do such a thing—and bill for doing it. Sig Hansen, the then world-renowned chief of orthopedics at HMC, taught the medics to put compound femur fracture in Thomas ring splints because he knew he was going to open them up, debride the wound, and start antibiotics anyhow. Early on, some physicians and hospitals in the community opposed most of this work on the grounds that it wasn't safe, but in reality, it was mostly about who would get the work.

In 1975, hospitals all over Seattle got together voluntarily and, under the auspices of the King County Medical Society, agreed to list what they were capable of receiving acutely: psychiatry, obstetrics, trauma, cardiac arrest, coma, and so forth. Theoretically, people were assigned to a hospital based on what that hospital itself had already said it could treat. In fact, the paramedics delivered all major trauma to Harborview because doctors and ancillary staff were always there, not simply on call but available somewhere in the building.

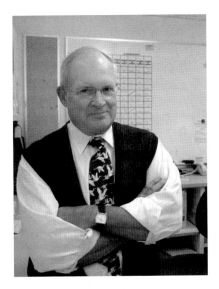

Dr. Copass in the Harborview "fish bowl," 1992. *Courtesy of Medic One.*

The turf battles were eventually settled because Medic One was working, the community hospitals all had plenty of trade, on-call doctors didn't have to get up at night, and the sickest patients got immediate attention at HMC. "There was a guy named William Weinstein, a cardiologist at the old Doctors Hospital, who was the brother of Dr. Copass's beloved high school math teacher," Ralph Maughn (a paramedic trained in group two) told some of his buddies after they'd taken a patient there. "The CCU at Doctors was one bed and a door, and Weinstein was standing next to a resident at the only bedside. 'Kid, there's one thing I want you to remember. If I drop right now here's what you do. I want you to pick up the phone, call 911, ask for Medic One, and get the hell outta the way,' he told the startled young resident."

Copass was a constant in the Harborview ED. But the resident staff rotated, so it was the nurses, of course, who really ran the triage, initiated care, took care of people, and—sometimes when it got too busy at night—even stitched them up. Chris Martin started there in 1976 as a young nurse with only two years' experience. She remembered that Mike Copass was already a towering figure by then, and "you shook in your boots if he started to ask you too many questions. But he also brought his kids in on some Saturday mornings, and put them in a corner of the fish bowl to color." On a July evening soon after Nurse Martin started, Anna Stevens, an RN for thirty years, was precepting her as she went to help a patient from the street get undressed to be examined and have his vital signs taken. "I was a middle-class kid, and Anna watched as I peeled off his pants down to his shoes, which were sopping. In my life, no one peed in their pants and filled up their shoes, so I asked him if it was raining outside. Anna stood in the hall laughing, and I realized then it was best if people took off their own shoes if they could."[36] Another of the things that made the Emergency Department function well through the 1970s and '80s was that Dr. Copass knew so many of the repeaters, where they hung out, and what was the matter with them. On occasion when a call came in to Medic One about someone found down at a certain intersection, he might say, "Oh, that could be bad. There's a bar on that corner, and a park across the street. That's where a guy I know named Eddie usually sleeps; he has congestive heart failure—and enemies."

No matter who was hauled in, however, Dr. Copass did whatever he could to make them feel important and safe. Chris Martin, who eventually became the administrative director of the ED and later of Airlift NW, said, "He brought people lying on a gurney warm blankets himself. He taught us all that the down and outers were just as important as the president of the United States, and he told people that." For these patients weren't bums or addicts or derelicts or gomers who happened to show up in the ER when Mike Copass was the director. Then they were known as "the unfortunates." It was also during these years that paramedics on the rigs learned that during their runs, both night and day, Dr. Copass was usually listening on his "Portable 55" radiophone to their conversations with the trauma doc who was their nominal control. Occasionally, as the medics and the second-year surgery resident were working out how to manage a problem, questions arose. Mick Oreskovich, who was one of the ED surgeons then (before he became a psychiatrist), remembers a conversation from the field when the medics were treating a patient with seizures they were having trouble stopping.[37] Fearing that they might lose the woman's airway, they asked permission to intubate her. The trauma doc told them instead to give more Valium, the first-line IV drug used to treat seizures in those years. The medics resisted, and again said they wanted to intubate her. Suddenly, over Portable 55 from the dark of his bedroom, came Copass's voice, hoarse from sleep: "push the Valium!" They immediately did, and the seizures immediately stopped. The paramedics repeat this story in many similar forms about a variety of situations.

As director of the ED, Dr. Copass possessed a special parking space adjacent to the hospital. This was a great perk for people with certain jobs because the HMC parking lots were often full even at night, and the big multistory one facing Puget Sound hadn't been expanded and was farther away. He had a series of old BMWs he worked on himself with more or less success, and as he was leaving one late fall night, the white one wouldn't start. He decided to take the #3 Metro bus downtown to Third and Pike, transfer to the Mercer Island bus, and get home. The street was empty and dark when he got off near what was then the downtown Bon Marché, and as he stood alone at the bus stop holding his always-present small doctor's bag full of neurology gear, three young toughs approached. They demanded his bag and wallet. Mike firmly said no and tried to reason with them. After a couple minutes of increasingly intense debate, one of the young men pulled a knife. Mike hauled up his radiophone and said, "Help the officer. Portable 55 needs assistance at Third and Pike." Within about thirty seconds, half of the cops in the downtown corridor were there, and within another minute almost all of them had screeched up. As the Mercer Island bus pulled to the curb, Dr. Copass stepped over the three handcuffed guys on the ground and calmly boarded. The fellow lying on his belly who had pulled the knife looked up at the police office standing above him and said, "Who's Portable 55?"[38]

5

DISARMING THE BOXES

T
here were a lot of false alarms," former firefighter Dick DeFaccio recalled when explaining why all the fire alarm boxes were removed from around the city.[39]

Years earlier, DeFaccio had entered the University of Washington intending to study commercial art, but after insulting a professor one day, he was invited to reconsider. "It was a life drawing class," he remembered, "and the professor spent the entire hour walking around the room looking at our work and saying things like, 'That line is unfortunate'—that was his favorite. He never offered help."

One morning, when his teacher repeated the by then intolerable remark to his student, DeFaccio unceremoniously asked, "What the hell does that mean anyway?" He was told to leave the room, but instead said, "Like hell I will. I'm paying to be here, and you're paid to teach. Now either do that, or *you* get out. As I recall, the rest of the students just kept their heads down and continued to work. There were several audible snickers from classmates." It was the sixties, after all.

The following morning, he was summoned from another class to the office of the dean, who simply asked, "Do you think you would prefer to pursue a different major?"

"By that time," the now retired DeFaccio remembered, "I was sure I would."

When he graduated with a business degree in 1968, he went to work for the family machining company on Harbor Island. "I'd been there about two years, but just as the Boeing economic slowdown got underway late in 1970, my older brother thought I wasn't doing an adequate job of selling, so he fired me. And I probably wasn't. It was hard to sell much then."

For a couple of years, he did a little of everything, including spending time as an electrician's helper pulling wires and selling wholesale electrical supplies to hardware stores. He also worked as doorman/bouncer at Embers Tavern on Alki. Then he applied to the fire department, though without much hope of acceptance because they had two thousand applicants and only eighty-three jobs for new recruits. But he was hired. He joined the largest class since World War II. "So big," DeFaccio remembered, "they divided us into two groups for training, one a night shift that started at 5:00 p.m. and finished at 3:00 a.m. The week our instruction began in late January of 1972, it snowed almost a foot in Seattle. Then it froze. The first week was hose training behind Station 14 at Forth and Horton and that, of course, froze. We could hardly stand. The work uniform for recruits was Penny's gray cotton shirt and pants, light blue jacket, oxford shoes, and a helmet." It was a little unusual then for a college grad like DeFaccio to be a fire recruit. Ed Prendergast, the chief of personnel who interviewed all the applicants after the initial testing, told Dick that he was overqualified. He proved that in a way when he finished first in the class.

For three years, DeFaccio worked in a combat division at Station 27 at Boeing Field. Like all rookies, he started on the tailboard and worked his way up to acting battalion lieutenant. Suddenly, in the spring of 1975,

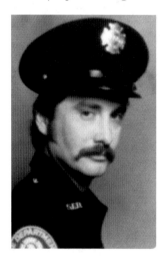

Owen Pletan, the chief of communications, asked DeFaccio to come down to the Alarm Center, then located on the grounds of Seattle Center near a simulated ICU used for training paramedics. Pletan, who knew DeFaccio as a recruit, had apparently been impressed by his intelligence, perseverance, and ingenuity.

By that time, Seattle had instituted basic 911, and the fire alarm boxes were more trouble than the upkeep was worth. "Pletan wanted me to write a proposal to the City Council Budget Office to eliminate the antiquated fire alarm boxes scattered around town because they were almost always false alarms, pranks, and seldom real fires. The department still had to respond, but it took units out of service, and it was troublesome."

Dick DeFaccio as twenty-seven-year-old firefighter in 1972. *Courtesy Richard DeFaccio.*

The alarm box system was old, outdated, used costly overhead copper wire, and was expensive to maintain. In the process of taking it down, DeFaccio discovered that the same wires also served other essential communications functions linked directly to the fire stations, and actually were necessary to set off their alarm bells. So Chief Pletan said, "Now write a proposal to upgrade the entire communications system."

The whole thing had grown archaic; it actually used telegraph keys to transmit some kinds of information. It was up to DeFaccio first to design a more modern analog system for dispatch and station communications. He first came up with a radiophone scheme that had backup power to both simplify and greatly improve the speed and reliability of transmitted information. In the end, he submitted a comprehensive design proposal to upgrade the whole infrastructure, including computer-assisted dispatch, new dispatcher consoles, and a digital Fire Alarm Center phone system.

Next, he had to convince the Budget Office to use the money being saved by not having to maintain the copper wire and the removed alarm box system (about $300,000 a year) to implement the improved system he

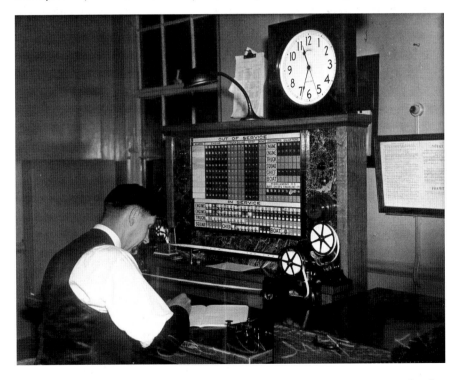

Old watch desk where signals from the firebox registered the box number, then correlated with the assignment cards. *Courtesy of Seattle Fire Department.*

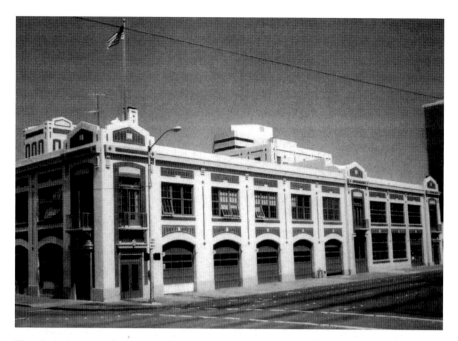

Fire alarm center station, 1961–91, at 408 Thomas Street. *Courtesy of Seattle Fire Department.*

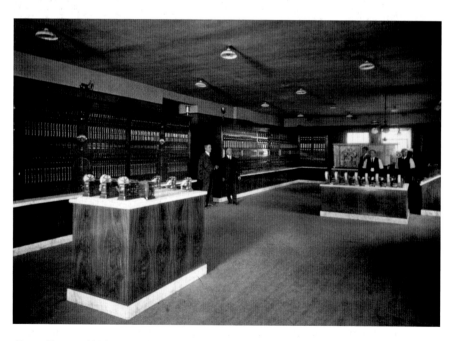

Alarm Center, 1912–25, at Station 10, Third Avenue South at Main. *Courtesy of Seattle Fire Department.*

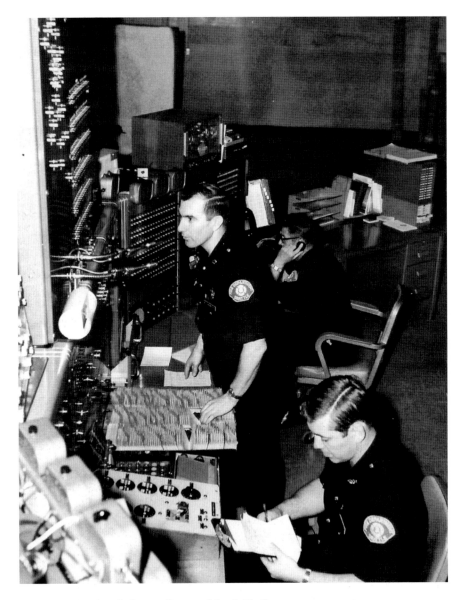

Firefighters locating the boxes. *Courtesy of Seattle Fire Department.*

had suggested. Finally, the fire department's budget analyst, Jack Raab, a tough negotiator, became convinced that the proposed new system would not only be cost neutral but would actually save some money in the future. In this way, the fire department redesigned its entire alarm center communications system.

By then, Renton had joined Seattle with the installation of basic 911, meaning that if a phone exchange was at least partly in Seattle, citizens could call 911 and get the cops. In practice, this meant that a call to 911 went to what was then termed the Public Safety Answering Point, meaning the police first. Then the dispatcher decided what department needed to respond and appropriately transferred the call by hand. This process was slow, cumbersome, and prone to errors.

In addition to slow analog equipment, a second obstruction was that the telephone exchange boundaries didn't match the fire and municipal boundaries, so there were a lot of misdirected calls. Prior to electronic switching, all calls had to be transferred manually to the correct agency. This required the dispatchers to know, for example, what part of the Cherry phone exchange was in Fire District 1, and what part of the Melrose exchange resided in Fire District 4. Due to this mismatch between telephone and jurisdictional boundaries, about 10 percent of those incoming calls were misdirected. Early on, this meant some very precious minutes went to figuring out even where people were when they called. By then, it was already very clear that if Medic One was to be successful, minutes counted.

From the start of 911, there was also a little controversy as to how and when a call should transfer to the fire department, because the police needed to know there wasn't a crime being committed in addition to a blaze or medical emergency. If the dispatcher determined it was purely a medical issue, they immediately transferred the call to the fire department, but if there was a possible crime in progress, that had to be negotiated in real time. DeFaccio described the process: "The police got fire on the line, but they continued to handle the interrogation until it was determined that the site was safe. There were always good relationships between fire, 911, and the police. They were a good group of guys, and we worked it out."

Another limitation of the basic 911 system was that it gave no exact location even if the boundaries in question were aligned. Dispatchers relied on the callers themselves to identify where they were. At the fire alarm center, that could be a traumatic experience: trying to figure out what the caller was saying when they were excited or terrified. DeFaccio recalled, "When I was there, we listened on two occasions while the caller burned to death because they couldn't give us a location. In both circumstances they were trapped."

The addition of Medic One added the tiered system of response to fire alarm calls. If the dispatcher felt that only Basic Life Support would most likely be required, he or she sent an engine company and aid car to the

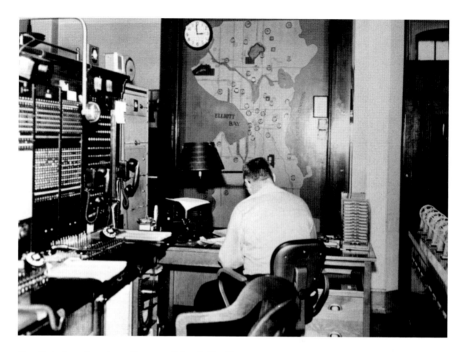

Pre-digital workstation. *Courtesy of Seattle Fire Department.*

scene. These responders then had the responsibility to decide whether or not they were capable of treating the injury themselves or if they needed Medic One. If the problem were purely medical, the dispatchers first asked, "Is the patient conscious?" and second, "Is the patient breathing?" When either answer was no, that patient was considered to be unstable, and the dispatcher immediately sent the paramedics. Medic One and the new communications system shaved off many valuable minutes between the call and onset of treatment. Dr. Cobb's data was proving that speed and well-trained paramedics saved lives.

Because of the success of the new system, DeFaccio stayed at the fire alarm center and became assistant to the chief of communications. Another firefighter, John Cushman, was working for a civilian financial officer analyzing what fire department resources were being dispatched under what circumstances. Part of their job was to understand fire responses, what people and equipment went to the scene, how long it took to get there, how long they stayed, and what the outcomes were. They used this data to develop algorithms for deciding what level of service was being provided under the existing protocols. Based on that information, they rebuilt this part of the

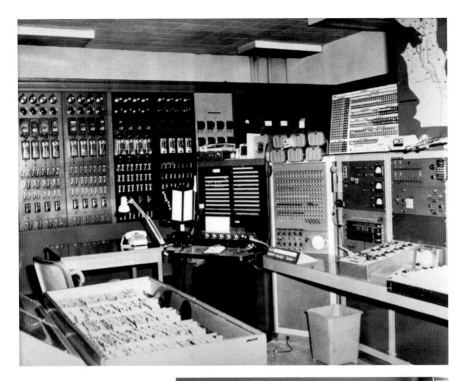

Above: File card box at pre-digital workstation. *Courtesy of Seattle Fire Department.*

Right: Alarm Center remnants of the pre-digital age. *Courtesy of Seattle Fire Department.*

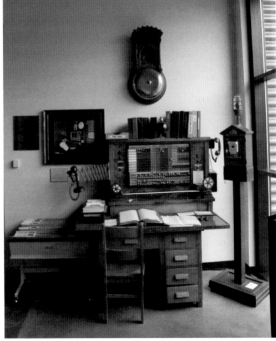

response system to pre-assign level of need and level of service indices to every intersection in the city. For example, if a fire was in a residential area, a full response was two engines, one ladder company, and one battalion chief. If it was in a downtown, industrial, or otherwise dense area, the response was much larger: five engines, two ladder companies, an attack unit, and two battalion chiefs.

At the same time this work was getting underway, DeFaccio designed a system for deploying uncommitted fire resources in the event of multiple-alarm fires. When the fire department was initially dispatched, whatever unit could get to an intersection first was known as the "first in." On arrival, the officer reported to the fire alarm center by radiophone what was happening on the ground and what might be needed beyond the personnel and equipment already there. A battalion chief arrived, took charge, and could amend or override the prior decisions. In the event of a multiple alarm fire, the new algorithm ensured that the entire city would still have adequate coverage. In those days, an engine with an EMS-trained firefighter always accompanied the run. However, in early 1975, there was only one Medic One rig and two other aid cars. Moby Pig was reassigned, probably now as someone's elaborate motor home, complete with built-in first aid.

When President Carter created FEMA by Executive Order in April 1979, he appointed Gordon Vickery to be the first acting director. John Cushman and DeFaccio proposed to Fire Chief Frank Hanson that, because of rapidly changing technology, he create a research and development section for the department. Hanson agreed. They had already developed basic computerized systems for distribution of resources, and the savvy Cushman thought they could get money from FEMA. They broadened the scope a little by proposing to modernize information technology jointly with the Portland Fire Department. Furthermore, to gain technical credibility, they partnered with Boeing computer services and applied to FEMA for a grant, which in spite of former Chief Vickery, they didn't get. They did, however, get funding to write a textbook about information technology for fire departments. They involved Phoenix, Salt Lake City, Los Angeles, and others in a development meeting to write the text, which Boeing published.

Using Seattle as the model, the book included a Level of Need and Level of Service index for every intersection in town. Initially printed on cards kept at the Alarm Center, these described what firehouse was to be the first response station for every location and then the order of escalation should things get worse. However, the information was

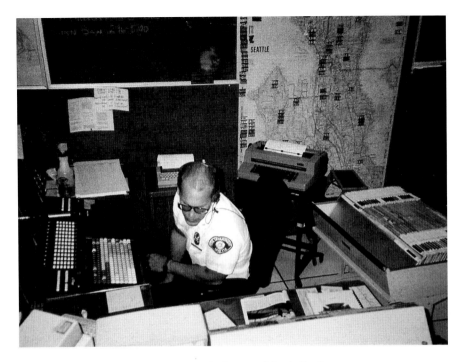

Fire alarm center at Station 2, 1991–2008. *Courtesy of Seattle Fire Department.*

constantly changing, and therefore the cards needed continual revision, a labor-intensive task. The algorithm was later computerized, allowing EMT firefighters and Medic One paramedics to arrive both faster and more reliably at the correct place.

When the fire department buildings at Seattle Center were removed, there was another upgrade and the Alarm Center went into an unused theater in Station 2. Much more sophisticated computers were then put in use. Now there is a new fire alarm center in its own building at Station 10 in Pioneer Square, where everything is localized by GPS. But vital signs still remain the trigger for what level of aid is sent. Dispatchers must continue to keep panicked people on the line in order to figure out that level of need. Dick DeFaccio remembered callers saying, "Send somebody, send somebody," and calm dispatchers replying, "I have somebody on the way, but I need more information. Don't hang up."

All of these systems were in place on February 2, 1989. One of the paramedics then assigned to the Medic One unit dispatched from Harborview recalled that a rare storm had blanketed the city with six inches of heavy snow earlier that night. Dozens of young people had taken to Seattle's streets, particularly the downhill ones emptied of traffic, and filled them up with sleds.

As Jerry Ehrler, one of those early paramedics dispatched to the scene of an accident that night, remembered, "That's when the calls started. The Fire Alarm Center described our patient as a fourteen-year-old female sledding downhill very fast who had collided with a parked vehicle. The intersection lay at the bottom of Queen Anne Hill. In 1989, the likelihood of finding a helmeted adolescent on a sled was slight. As we feared, she had struck the steel fender of a sedan headfirst. Due to the difficult road conditions, Engine 41 got to the location a few minutes before we did. The crew had placed a rigid collar around the child's neck and positioned her on a backboard to protect her spinal column. They were having difficulty finding a pulse or recording blood pressure. There was obvious external evidence of a traumatic brain injury."[40] In a very short time, she arrested. But clinically dead in Seattle, even in 1989, was treatable, and they did treat her. Her young heart responded. Soon she had a pulse, blood pressure, and breath, so they turned on the lights and sped hopefully to Harborview.

For a while on the way, her vital signs remained stable. But as the paramedics examined the extent of her injury and monitored her neurological exam, hope faded. By the time they reached the ED, the injury seemed almost certainly fatal. Later, when the senior paramedic sat down to write the report required for every patient, he identified the child as twelve-year-old Karen Maleng, daughter of Norm Maleng, popular longtime King County prosecutor. Jerry Ehrler is now the education coordinator for the Medic One Paramedic Training Program. Seventeen years later, that night remained vivid in his memory:

> *After completing the form and leaving a copy with Harborview staff, I stepped into the hallway and saw the very recognizable figure of Norm Maleng walking toward me. In my Seattle Fire Department uniform, I too was identifiable. There was no one else around. It seemed to me that I was to be the one to give Mr. Maleng the worst of news. The distance between us was shrinking quickly, and I was more and more uncomfortable. When he was no more than twenty feet away, a door on my right opened silently and Dr. Copass appeared. With his always graceful compassion, he told Mr. Maleng that his daughter would die. The entire team so impressed Judy and Norm Maleng that, eventually containing their grief, they became leading advocates and allies for Medic One and the Trauma Center at Harborview.[41]*

In 2000, the voters of King County approved a $193 million bond measure to construct the Maleng Building at 410 Ninth Avenue across the street from the Harborview Emergency Department entrance. The top floor of that building houses the new HMC Trauma ICU.

Can paramedics be taught to do a lot of what doctors do?

Absolutely. But citizens learned that lesson more easily and faster in some American cities than in others.

6

THE TREATMENT OF
NEGLECTED DISEASES

B y the late 1960s, Seattle and the Pacific Northwest were not the only
places in the United States where doctors, firefighters, and politicians
were discovering the promise of pre-hospital care. Following the
work Pantridge had done in Belfast, the National Research Council of
the National Academy of Sciences joined the discussion in 1966, thus
involving the U.S. federal government. That year, the Academy published an
influential white paper titled "Accidental Death and Disability: the Neglected
Diseases of Modern Society."[42] This forty-four-page document concluded
with a list of recommendations that not only summarized plans to enhance
training in advanced first aid for rescue personnel, including ambulance
attendants, police, and firefighters, but also offered an outline for what was
to become a broad national emergency medicine system. Eventually, the
effort incorporated the entirety of training and regulation for personnel,
communications, transportation, facilities, and registries documenting the
treatment of injured people.

Over several years, public interest in these services grew, and jurisdictions
from coast to coast (even extending to Hawaii) tried to figure out ways to
either incorporate pre-hospital care into existing structures and budgets or
ways to design new ones.

The public health implications of the National Academy of Sciences
findings were significant. In the year 1965 alone, 52 million Americans
had been seriously hurt, 10 million of them at least temporarily impaired,
and more than 400,000 permanently disabled. An additional 107,000

people died of their injuries.[43] To alleviate these disabilities, deaths, and the staggering $18 billion yearly cost to society, Lyndon Johnson formed the Presidential Commission on Highway Safety, and Congress soon passed the National Highway Safety Act of 1966, providing funds. In 1973, Congress overrode a Richard Nixon veto and passed the Emergency Medical Services Act authorizing the Department of Health, Education, and Welfare to award $160 million in regional grants over three years to enhance EMS across the country.

Not surprisingly, cities, counties, and states quickly lined up to apply for the money. By 1975, more than two hundred grants had been awarded. No longer would patients be deposited in emergency rooms and wait for junior house officers to search them out on gurneys in remote corners. All over America, the emergency room was going out to find the sick and injured people where they fell.

Relieved of McCarthy-era risks of having the communist stigma nailed to them, public health officials and departments had become much more proactive. Rather than the traditional behavioral intervention model, public health interventions for injury control began to include identifying causative agents, mitigating the agents and the activity of the agents, and improving emergency, definitive, and rehabilitative care. The attitude was also reflected in comments made by George E. Pickett, MD, a member of the Executive Board of the American Public Health Association during Senate testimony. Pickett stated,

> *The health professional has a growing major role in the development of research, education, environmental modification, and emergency care to prevent and ameliorate injury, disability, and economic loss from accidents. Proposed and promoted improvements in EMS followed this belief, as reflected in the media. The lay press reported these advances and reported many individual cases of patients being brought back to life.*[44]

James Page was one of those public health officials. Like Pantridge in Ireland and Cobb in Seattle, Page was an influential early champion of pre-hospital care to deliver emergency medical services. From firsthand experience, he also championed improved organization. He had begun his career as a firefighter in Monterey Park, California, and rose to become a battalion chief in Los Angeles. As is the case with many visionary people, he promoted his own beliefs. Colleagues noted that he was good at it because, "he had the gumption to express these ideas through whatever medium presented itself, be it a TV show, a magazine, a conference, a public meeting, a book, a video, or an official report." Also an attorney, Page was an effective public advocate for the statewide emergency medical systems he had helped to organize in California, North Carolina, and New York. But it was perhaps his role as the technical advisor to the television program *Emergency* first aired in 1972 that helped to fix his place in history. Viewers loved the popular singer, actress, and former pinup model Julie London as nurse Dixie McCall and paramedic Johnny Gage, whose character is considered by many to have been based on the experiences of Jim Page.

Page's other significant contribution was research he conducted on public policy with regard to the training and organization of the disparate paramedic programs emerging in the late 1960s. His report, published as *The National Study of Paramedic Law and Policy* by Lakes Area Emergency Medical Services (1976), noted that more than half of the existing programs had been established without state legislation. In fact, between 1969 and 1975, twenty-five states established paramedic programs with no legal authority. In addition, Page claimed, there were not even agreed-upon names for either the programs or the participants.[45]

Nonetheless, several cities and states continued to reply to the vigorous public demand for these services, including down the West Coast from Seattle.

LOS ANGELES

The year after Len Cobb first stopped in to see Gordon Vickery, two programs aimed at establishing EMS departments arose in Los Angeles. But in the City of Angels, antagonism distinguished the efforts, and in spite of Jim Page's lobbying, this competition delayed any real implementation of a comprehensive program in the region by several years.

In late 1969, at the Daniel Freeman Memorial Hospital in Inglewood (since sold and renamed Centinela Freeman Regional Medical Center, Memorial Campus), cardiologist Walter Graf began organizing a plan to train paramedics that survived until 1972.[46] Although supported by the LA County Heart Association and other local community hospitals, the effort lacked infrastructure. Dr. Graf and his colleagues did succeed in designing and equipping a dedicated coronary care ambulance, and a team that included trained Coronary Care Unit nurses, but there were too few resident doctors available twenty-four hours a day to enable a swift and coherent physician-directed response to cardiac crises. After an on-call physician eventually initiated dispatch, their step van truck converted into an ambulance lumbered to the nearest of the three participating hospitals, picked up a CCU nurse, and only then drove to the scene. This cumbersome system was as slow as the early Pantridge schemes, and even after the addition of paramedics, it ultimately was abandoned by the hospital.

The other program was stationed at Harbor General Hospital, a seven-hundred-bed teaching center affiliated with the UCLA Medical School. It was better staffed, better funded, and finally more successful. Though the LA Fire Department had equipped all its vehicles with basic first aid equipment about the same time Seattle Fire did, like Washington State, California lacked any legislation that would permit paramedics to operate independently.

Nonetheless, in September 1969, J. Michael Criley and A. James Lewis, curiously both cardiologists who must not have cared for their first names, inaugurated the paramedic training program at Harbor General. The initial class of eighteen firefighters included twelve from LA County and six from the city. Carol Bebout, an experienced CCU nurse, and Dr. Criley supervised their 180 hours of instruction, and by December of that year, the first ACLS paramedics went to work in LA.[47] The requirement that the rigs be supervised by on-board medical doctors still hampered the program.

Graf, a canny politician, recruited Kenneth Hann to help push through legislation in Sacramento that would legally permit paramedics to work independently. Hann, a longtime member of the LA County Board of Supervisors, proposed a bill that passed as the Wedworth-Townsend Paramedic Act in 1970. Through an affiliation with El Camino Community College District, the LA County Health Services Paramedic Training Institute enhanced its standing as an academic program by providing college credit.[48]

SAN DIEGO

Farther south, and perhaps without the Hollywood glamor and certainly with no TV show, emergency medical management had been the responsibility of the San Diego Police Department. They had little training and less equipment. In 1972, the City of San Diego won part of the HEW Special Projects Grants as a demonstration undertaking. In cooperation with the UCSD Medical Center, the county introduced successful training programs (like Los Angeles, at local community colleges) and was subsequently able to establish proof of principle that EMS saved lives. Even so, the community didn't buy it.

When San Diego Fire proposed taking over pre-hospital care in 1975, the chief wanted to impose a new tax to pay for the service. That effort went to a vote of the people, who soundly defeated the plan. A committee to resolve the issue recommended that a private ambulance company take charge. For some unnamed political reason, this decision was immediately reversed, and the subsequent battle between public and private management of EMS in San Diego took years to resolve.

In 1979, the city finally settled on a two-tiered system similar to the one adopted in Seattle, employing both BLS private ambulance services for routine calls and ALS Fire Department–trained paramedics for life-threatening trauma. But because of long response times, especially in rural areas, even that wasn't the end of the squabble. In 1997, the city addressed this regional deficiency when San Diego Fire joined with the local Rural Metro agencies to form the organization now called San Diego Medical Services Enterprise. Replacing the competition with cooperation, both the logistics of the entire operation as well as the outcomes for patients improved.

Cooperation also began to produce data in San Diego, and the real advances in medicine are largely data-driven. A significant contribution arrived in 2003 when the San Diego paramedics published a prospective study reporting a three-year experience with rapid sequence intubation. This technique bypasses some traditional, slower steps in placing an endotracheal tube into patients at high risk for aspiration. In a patient with a belly full of food or drink, or one who has already vomited, fluids from the oral pharynx might bypass the esophagus and enter the lungs. By sedating and paralyzing such patients with short-acting drugs, the San Diego group proved they could be safely intubated immediately. This practice is now widely accepted in specific emergency situations.[49]

HONOLULU

In Hawaii, the pace of life at the time was slower than on the mainland. EMS was also slower to be adopted and took some quirky turns to get there. Four young men led by ambulance attendant Bryan Peterson moved to the islands from California in 1969 and, with very little standing in their new community, formed the American Paramedical Institute Inc. Through this vehicle, they hoped to evaluate and improve emergency care in Honolulu (as well as to establish themselves). They had no experience in such a venture—and no money—but with the exuberance of the young, they began to raise both the necessary cash and the sought-after notice by holding a rock concert fundraiser followed by an international conference. The concert at the Diamond Head Volcano benefit raised a little money, and the conference raised some eyebrows.[50]

With the $7,000 collected by asking for donations from the crowd, Institute founders began their evaluation of the Honolulu ambulances, equipment, and training. The report that followed publicly criticized the establishment, and Mayor Frank Fasi didn't like it. Neither did most of the other local officials. Undeterred, the young Institute founders sent out invitations to health officials in the United States, Europe, Russia, Israel, China, South Africa, and Australia inviting them to attend the First International Symposium on EMS. When letters of acceptance began to arrive by the bagful, organizers found themselves unprepared financially, as well as woefully inexperienced in the protocols and diplomacy necessary for hosting such a gathering. "Should Arabs and Israelis be seated at the same banquet table? Should Russians or the Chinese get top billing on the program?" Nobody knew.[51]

Neither, at that rebellious societal moment, did any of the transplanted California organizers own a necktie. Bryan Peterson, the dominant Institute planner, therefore issued a proclamation that banned ties at the conference, surprising the British delegates. The State Department too was alarmed, not because of the ban on neckties but because of the arrival of the international secretary of the Soviet Medical Workers Union at the meeting.

In advance of the gathering, the Institute distributed its negative findings about local emergency services. That error, combined with the Hawaii Medical Association's discounted prior efforts to improve EMS in the islands, caused the physicians' group to boycott the conference. The governor of the State of Hawaii, who had been invited by the organizers to deliver opening remarks at the conference, declined. Instead, he sent the lieutenant governor, who didn't show up, and the First International Symposium on EMS was also the last act of the American Paramedical Institute Inc.

The Hawaiian Medical Association, however, accelerated its efforts to improve training. By 1971, two hundred hours of didactic education plus two hundred hours of supervised clinical experience were required to become an ambulance attendant. Because of the scattered geography of the state, which includes eight major islands and dozens of smaller ones, transportation of major trauma or cardiac victims by water was often too late. Helicopters had a much better record, and in 1974, the U.S. Army 68th Medical Detachment began emergency transportation through a system eventually known as Military Assistance to Safety and Traffic (MAST). These pilots saved civilian lives in many settings until 1982, when the program was halted because of a perceived overlap with private enterprise.

By 1975, under sponsorship of the State Medical Society, paramedics began to be certified in Hawaii. Honolulu Fire took over the direction of first responders in 1976. As happened in many jurisdictions in the 1980s, paramedic education moved to community college instructors.

••••

Across the continent, three other American cities embraced paramedic education early and with the same vigor as had the founders of the program in Seattle. These disparate sites were Columbus, Ohio; Pittsburgh, Pennsylvania; and Miami, Florida.

COLUMBUS

In 1931, an unknown citizen donated a now equally unknown device called a Lyons pulmotor (a primitive kind of pressure-regulated ventilator) to the Columbus Fire Department. Patented in 1921 by Edward H. Lyon of Cleveland, this contraption looked like a large bicycle pump. It was equipped with a mask to be placed over the victim's nose and mouth, connected by two hoses permitting an operator to force a mixture of room air and oxygen under pressure into the lungs.[52] Although it could be dangerous (because it might force material from the mouth into the lungs) and didn't work very well (because it was basically a bicycle pump), for some years, the chief carried it around in the back of his car. Thus, the pulmotor is remembered as the beginning of pre-hospital care in that city.

The next step was the Columbus "Heartmobile," a student design project at the University of Cincinnati that looked frighteningly like Seattle's Moby Pig. It worked a little better. Like Seattle's first effort, the Heartmobile was a modern ambulance only in the sense that it carried medical personnel and equipment. The principle advantage of this vehicle rebuilt on a mobile home chassis over the traditional ambulance of the day was a larger workspace,

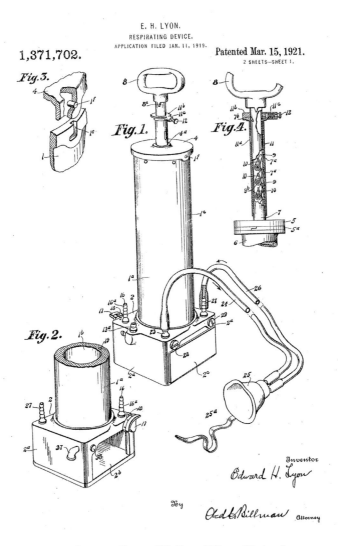

E. H. LYON.
RESPIRATING DEVICE.
APPLICATION FILED JAN. 11, 1919.

1,371,702.

Patented Mar. 15, 1921.
2 SHEETS—SHEET 1.

Fig. 3.

Fig. 1.

Fig. 4.

Fig. 2.

Inventor
Edward H. Lyon

By

Ord & Billman *Attorney*

Lyons Pulmotor patent diagram. *Courtesy U.S. Patent Office, public domain.*

allowing a patient to be placed in the vehicle on a stretcher and the staff to stand on both sides.

In 1968, Dr. James Warren was chair of the Department of Medicine at The Ohio State University School of Medicine. At about the same time undergrads designed the Heartmobile, Warren won a regional grant to start a pre-hospital coronary care service modeled on the one in Belfast. The Heartmobile hit the streets in 1969. Initially staffed by a cardiologist and three off-duty Columbus firefighters, it was dispatched in response to emergency cardiac events that were called in to the cardiologist. By 1971, when Columbus Fire took over EMS management, those same firefighters formed the core of the first class of paramedics and began to function without their previously required physician supervision. Response times, as well as outcomes, improved. By 1975, medics initially treated 55 percent of all heart attacks within the city of Columbus.[53]

Jim Warren became a believer in pre-hospital care and said so to the country on the *Today Show* when he explained that paramedics were both effective and relatively inexpensive in providing expert pre-hospital care in Columbus.[54]

Currently, in the state of Ohio there are twenty-seven community and technical colleges that offer courses leading to certification as an EMT or paramedic.

PITTSBURGH

As filmmaker and Hollywood paramedic Gene Starzenski, who grew up in Pittsburgh, remembered in a 2015 NPR story,

> *In the 1960s, Pittsburgh, like most cities, was segregated by race. But people of all colors suffered from lack of ambulance care. Police were the ones who responded to medical emergency calls. Back in those days, you had to hope and pray you had nothing serious, because basically, the only thing they did was pick you up and threw you in the back like a sack of potatoes, and they took off for the hospital. They didn't even sit in the back with you.*[55]

Then came Freedom House Enterprises. Following the assassination of Martin Luther King in 1968, riots broke out in urban neighborhoods all over America, including the Hill District in Pittsburgh. Freedom House, a nonprofit founded to foster African American businesses in the city, partnered with Phillip Hallen, then director of the Maurice Falk Medical Fund, a foundation attempting to bring healthcare to poor people. "No one would go to the Hill District, in the same way that taxicabs were hesitant to go there," said Hallen.[56]

"Blacks were not the only Pittsburgh residents who suffered from lack of care in those days. In 1966, the city's mayor collapsed. By the time he reached the hospital in a police car, he had gone too long without oxygen; he later died."[57] However, the Hill District African Americans were the first to actually try to do something about it. Phil Hallen was a former ambulance driver, and on the advice of a social worker, he began to envision a program to train unemployed black men and women to be medical technicians. That's when Hallen approached Freedom House. He sought help from Dr. Peter Safar, chair of the Department of Anesthesia at the University of Pittsburgh, who had designed the first medical intensive care program and was an early advocate for modern CPR.[58] The Freedom House Ambulance Service began to train people from the community in 1967 and, following three hundred hours of didactic study and nine months of clinical education in hospitals and on-board ambulances, the next year they started to transport and care for patients themselves.

They ran smack into the traditional Pittsburgh Police Department, which also operated an ambulance service. Obstructed both by shaky funding and by the cops, Freedom House took several years and a pile of collected data to become successful. "A 1971 study found that 62 percent of patients received inappropriate care from the police, while 11 percent received inappropriate care from Freedom House. Eventually, police officers in need of an ambulance for themselves or a family member would call the Freedom House dispatcher instead of the police."[59]

Dr. Nancy Caroline became the medical director, and "In 1975, Freedom House paramedics presented a disaster drill for an international symposium on critical care medicine. They were judged among the most sophisticated and skilled in the nation."[60] But that was also the year the city ended its contract with Freedom House, and Pittsburgh Fire took over management of EMS.

Today, with some pride, the fire department notes that it provides

> pre-hospital emergency medical care to the sick and injured citizens and guests of the 88 neighborhoods in the City of Pittsburgh. It is not uncommon for our ambulances to answer several hundred calls for service in any twenty-four-hour period. According to recent statistics we receive roughly one hundred seventy-eight calls per day! Along with the emergency treatment and transport of patients, the Ambulance Division is also responsible for providing medical coverage for special events throughout the City of Pittsburgh. From neighborhood functions to large events like the G20 Summit in 2009, paramedics are present at a large variety of special events.[61]

Freedom House Enterprises should be remembered gratefully for its early contributions.

MIAMI

In a 2015 talk to the staff at the University of Florida Department of Emergency Medicine, EMS pioneer Dr. Eugene Nagel said of early EMS in the region, "In those days ambulances carried 3 things: bandages, oxygen and splints, and they only charged for oxygen and for mileage just like a taxi."[62] An anesthesiologist at the University of Miami, Nagel practiced at Jackson Memorial Hospital. Like Harborview in Seattle, Harbor General in LA and other Level 1 major trauma centers affiliated with medical schools, Jackson Memorial manages injuries from all over the region and provides a majority of care to the underserved.

Because he was first trained as an electrical engineer and learned early resuscitation techniques as a resident at Columbia, Dr. Nagel's expertise in anesthesia merged with CPR. He was therefore a local expert and, in 1964, spoke at the International First Aid and Rescue Association meeting held in Miami. "I don't even remember what I talked about," he said. "And I was surrounded by a large number of equally befuddled doctors talking about bone injuries, this injury and that injury—talking to a group of largely lay-people who had absolutely no authority to do things like set splints and so on."[63] After that meeting, Nagel began to teach basic CPR to firefighters and came to admire and befriend them.

He soon became convinced that the state of the art was abysmal, techniques for cardiac resuscitation were primitive, and though he was not aware of Frank Pantridge, he concluded independently that "the only way to save cardiac arrest victims was to have firefighters defibrillate at the scene."[64] However, the Miami Fire chief was not as interested in that idea as Gordon Vickery had been in Seattle. In fact, said Dr. Nagel, "His apprehensions were apparent from the beginning. It was clear he had deep reservations about going too far." He wanted his department to look good and feared failure. Dr. Nagel remembered a meeting at which he explained to the chief that he hoped to teach his firefighters defibrillation. "A big, tall, 6'3" Irishman by the name of Lawrence Kenny, he had been quite tolerant of me up to now. He took his finger and he punched me in the chest and drove me back about three feet with that one finger." Kenny kept that up, while repeating to the much less bulky anesthesiologist, "This is a fire department, not a hospital; these are firemen and not doctors. I don't want you to forget that."[65]

But Eugene Nagel did forget it. At about the same time when Leonard Cobb did, he read the Frank Pantridge 1967 *Lancet* articles. Like Cobb, Nagel saw the solution to sudden cardiac death in the form of pre-hospital care. His main contribution to the advancement over Partridge's beginning was not his battle with the fire chief about paramedics but the addition of EKG telemetry.

With the help of a $3,000 grant from the Florida Heart Association, Nagel set out to develop a system capable of transmitting EKG over telephone lines. Such a new venture "seemed unlikely to hurt the patient or embarrass the department," Nagel assured the chief.[66] With his usual reluctance, Kenny agreed. The Biocom Company came up with a Motorola Business Dispatcher radio powered by a nickel-cadmium battery and married to a modulator, all "shock-mounted in an aluminum waterproof case to bring the whole unit to a backbreaking fifty-four pounds."[67] The device, while more substantial than portable, was nonetheless soon transmitting EKG tracings from afar to Dr. Nagel at Jackson Memorial. His next step in convincing the Miami Fire chief and city officials to train paramedics to provide independent treatment in the field required even more audacity. "I enlisted one of our residents, Harry Heinitsch," Nagel remembered.

> *Harry was the perfect candidate for me to ask since he enjoyed scuba diving to extreme depths, jumping out of planes, and other ways to endanger his life. So why not cater to his obvious death wish? We sprayed each other with topical anesthetic. I then intubated Harry, awake, demonstrating the technique. All nine paramedics then intubated Harry successfully. Harry then intubated me and the paramedics followed his lead.[68]*

This dramatic demonstration, which must have required more than a little bravado, not to mention tolerance for physical suffering, won permission from the City of Miami for physician-supervised paramedics to intubate in the field. Eugene Nagel went on to chair the Department of Anesthesia at Harbor General and to serve on the medical advisory committee to the International Association of Fire Chiefs.

Today, the City of Miami notes,

> *In addition to traditional fire services, firefighter/paramedics provide emergency medical care to victims of fires, accidents and sudden illnesses. Their ability to respond within four minutes helps save hundreds of lives each year and limits disabling injuries for the victims. The firefighter/ paramedic uses a sophisticated telemetry system that produces both voice and EKG transmission via radio. Personnel in this division staff fire stations strategically located throughout Miami's thirty-four square miles.[69]*

. . . .

All across the country, more jurisdictions applied for funds and sought better ways to provide organized, efficient, and rapid emergency care to patients at the scene. Tampa expanded its system from responding to fewer than three hundred emergency calls in 1955 to nearly thirteen thousand calls two decades later. Dallas sent EMT-trained firefighters on calls all over the city by 1972, and so did New York City, Birmingham, Alabama, and Bethesda, Maryland. Ten years later, most American cities had begun to require EMT certification as a condition of employment in their fire departments, and by May 2013, there were 237,660 EMTs and paramedics employed by local governments and other ambulance services in America.[70]

7

TEACHING HIGH SCHOOL GRADS
TO THINK LIKE DOCTORS

A fire department is a military-like operation, organized with rigorous command and control, which is perhaps why former soldiers Cobb and Copass liked it, and no doubt a big part of why the firefighters so liked them. By 1975, Medic One had two vehicles in operation, Al Alvarez had moved to Wyoming to be a cardiologist, and Dr. Copass had taken charge of training twenty-two students in the third class of paramedics. He had tried to get the community colleges to take on their classroom education, as had been done successfully elsewhere, but the administrators were reluctant to involve themselves too closely with the university.

After their first three hundred hours in the classroom, the paramedics' educations moved into what is still called the field internship. This phase included evaluation by both doctors and senior paramedics. Washington State law, which licensed the paramedics, is an exception to the physicians practice act and requires that there must be a mechanism for providing supervision. So Copass supervised the volunteer MD supervisors who rode the rigs.

Classroom training was initially organized in blocks: cardiac and pulmonary physiology, general medicine, neurology and coma, trauma, general surgery, and a general block that went into topics such as pediatrics, obstetrics, orthopedics, psychiatry, and neurosurgery. In addition to Copass, the early faculty included Dwayne Beatz, Greg Luna, Eileen Bulger, and Hugh Foy, who taught basic courses in the specifics

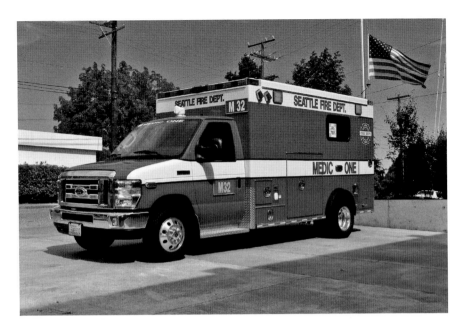

Medic One rig, late 1970s. *Courtesy of Seattle Fire Department.*

and all helped manage the general topics together. More senior UW faculty taught students how to treat the most subspecialized segments, such as facial fractures and burns.

Initially, the total period of their training was three months. But then came a push for state or national accreditation, and at a session of an AMA meeting in Chicago concerning various technical certifications, Dr. Copass first learned about the National Registry. This organization grew into a business for certifying paramedics that requires class time, hospital time, field time, and then passing a certifying test given by the National Registry company. A national certificate allows paramedics movement from place to place and state to state. Founded in 1970, the National Registry of Emergency Medical Technicians has its headquarters in Columbus, Ohio, also home of the original Heartmobile.

Before the new additions, Harborview paramedic training classes were originally held on the third floor of the hospital in the old neurology ward. The faculty bought a programmable mannequin that could be configured to represent various disease states and, depending on the variables, could be intubated, have IVs inserted, and display simulated EKG rhythms. Students pretended the dummy was a patient with one of a variety of problems they could work up. In 1972, after the World's Fair, the fire department built a simulated ICU in the Cascade rooms at Seattle Center, which for many years also included the Alarm Center. Here each student was responsible for overseeing the management of several simulated mannequin cardiac arrests, including transport under senior supervision.

Students also made hospital rounds and, when they weren't riding one of the rigs, worked in the ED. There also was an animal lab where they put dogs into ventricular fibrillation electrically and then performed canine resuscitation. The faculty taught them to do cricothyroidotomy on dogs and pigs in the event that a patient could not be intubated in the field.

Cobb, Copass, and the rest of the faculty had a goal of teaching the medics how to think through the probable illnesses and then put them into a situation where they had to problem solve very quickly. If they didn't do it properly, they got the dreaded "SEE ME" on the top of their test sheet. Dr. Copass chewed them out when he thought they deserved it and reassured them if they needed it. They talked about medicine. The students sometimes trembled, but all of them remembered the lessons and teased him about it later.

Then they were qualified for "third man time." Two students worked together, and a senior medic evaluated them on their teamwork. Could they assess a patient, control the crowd, manage the engine company, intubate, get IVs in, and so on? They had to pass a six-page evaluation with at least an 85 percent. When successful, they graduated to the formal internship and rode the rigs first with a senior medic, and then both the medic and a doctor evaluated the fireman student. The senior medics were much tougher on them than the doctors.

As a continuing education opportunity for all the paramedics, Copass then started a weekly afternoon and evening refresher course. Initially held on Wednesdays, this interfered with union activity and so became the Tuesday Series for Continuing Education, which continues today and is a requirement for recertification.

After Dr. Copass retired, David Carlbom assumed his functions as the director of the Michael K. Copass Paramedic Training Program at Harborview. He reports to William Bremner, now the longtime chair of the Department of Medicine in the UW School of Medicine. As a resident himself, Bremner rode the rigs and became an advocate for Medic One paramedics. Carlbom wryly suggests that his boss may have been one of the residents who taught the medics bad habits, such as putting in subclavian central venous lines (because of the risk of producing a pneumothorax or infection), though those habits are more often attributed to Pat Fleet, Len Hudson, and Mike Copass.

Dave Carlbom began his career as a volunteer with the Bainbridge Island Fire Department while he was still in high school:

In 1989, I was an eighteen-year-old volunteer firefighter about to start at Whitman College, and the Chief assigned me to drive Copass back to the ferry in a Fire Department Suburban after a drill. On the way to the ferry dock, I asked him if I could become a paramedic. He muttered something I didn't understand, so I said "what?" He told me to pull over and I thought, "Oh God, I hit somebody." I stopped, put it in park, and set the brake. I'm now freaking out, heart rate of 140, and sweating. He thought for a minute and then says "No, you can't be a paramedic. You have to go to medical school. There are thousands of people you haven't yet met who are waiting to meet you. You have to be a doctor." Then I drove on down to the ferry.

Dr. Carlbom, now UW associate professor of medicine in the Division of Pulmonary and Critical Care, said, "I don't know what he saw in me, and I was overwhelmed."[71]

Arguing now with the confidence of his predecessor, Dr. Carlbom asserted,

Our model is unique. Most of the training around the country is community college based. You graduate from high school, you're nineteen, good with your hands, and not ready for college. Your counselor says you should go learn to be a paramedic. So in most programs you go do 800 to 850 hours of class, then work with a preceptor for a month in a local ED, see some patients, start some IVs, then are supervised by a field-training officer while you see between 30 and 50 patients total. You intubate one or two humans, graduate, have a certificate, and go find a job. But these people are nineteen, aren't sure of what they are doing, lose interest, and so they don't work as paramedics long but find their path to become something else. Our model is different. Instead of a sequential process of class and training, we believe in a parallel process of progressive responsibility, and much more intensive training.[72]

Admission to paramedic training at Harborview is now closed, meaning only people who have a guaranteed job by their sponsoring agency, plus five years' experience as an EMT, are eligible. In an effort to get the best candidates, Dr. Carlbom and his staff provide coaching and counseling to the agencies and join them in interviewing the candidates if asked. Training is about 500 hours of classroom; 500 hours of laboratory; 1,500 hours training and experience in the HMC Emergency Department, ICU, OR, and clinics; and finally 1,500 hours in the field. The lab experience with programmable mannequins is supplemented by using pigs to learn cricothyrotomies. This procedure requires an incision in the cricothyroid membrane of the trachea to establish an emergency airway in a patient who cannot be intubated.

"Despite occasional pressure from animal rights groups," Dr. Carlbom said, "we think it is the best model to teach paramedics to save human beings. Physicians learn on humans, paramedics don't have that opportunity to learn about tissue and blood, so they learn on animals operated upon under general anesthesia and cared for by our vet."[73] The pig is going to become pork anyhow, one way or another.

Their field training starts right away on the second day when "they are not much use except to carry stuff," Dr. Carlbom said. Paramedic students first observe senior medics and then gradually assume more responsibility. When they finish, students have a three-part evaluation: an instructor assessment of individual skills, a senior paramedic evaluation of everything they do, and a physician assessment of what they have learned at the end. "The MDs," Dave Carlbom repeated, "are still not nearly as hard on them as the paramedics."

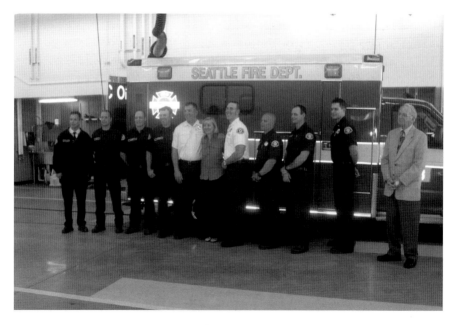

Len Cobb (*far right*), paramedics Zachary Drathman (*center left*) and Bryan Smith (*center right*), and firefighters outside Harborview about 2005. The woman between the paramedics had been resuscitated and saved by them. *Courtesy of Medic One.*

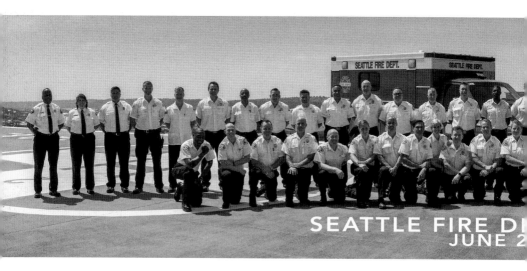

Seattle paramedics, June 2017. *Courtesy of Seattle Fire Department.*

Paramedic training at Harborview today requires about three thousand hours total. The field internship is ten intensive months long. Students each see about six hundred patients in the field, intubate forty-five human beings (thirty in OR and fifteen in the field), start 325 to 450 IVs, put in five to ten central lines, manage fifteen cardiac arrests themselves, and are the "in charge" medic for about three hundred patients. They work as sort of old-fashioned medical interns and are reviewed on every decision, and like old-school medical and surgical interns, they receive a lot of negative feedback.

Using this model since 1969, about 680 paramedics have been trained, and more than 200 of them remain in Seattle. In the fall of 2015, 24 more students began their study in the forty-second HMC paramedic class.

But they won't be done when they graduate. Medics are required to attend continuing education to be relicensed, so the Tuesday Series, initially started by Dr. Copass on Wednesdays in a classroom on that old HMC neurology ward, continues. They have an Advanced Cardiac Life Support (ACLS) refresher airway lab every two years and one hundred hours of Pediatric Advanced Life Support (PALS) training.

"What makes our model unique," Dave Carlbom noted, "are the three branches: very senior UW School of Medicine volunteer teachers, institutional support from HMC where the students are treated as members of the staff in the ED, and the fire department because they

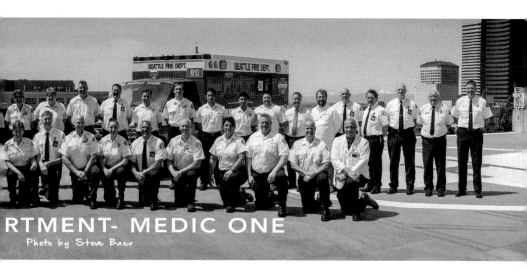

RTMENT- MEDIC ONE
Photo by Steve Baer

provide so much field training and teaching not only in the classroom but in the truck."[74] After every run, it is common for the medics to spend up to thirty minutes debriefing the student. The Medic One Foundation supports student tuition, so the department doesn't have to pay that, but it does pay indirectly to backfill the absence of the students when they aren't at the firehouse working, which is expensive.

Though the main focus for the early paramedics was cardiac, they have more recently been doing the same things for trauma. Using fellow EMTs as the victims, the students moulage them (*moulage* is French for casting, so the word means the art of cosmetically applying mock injuries for the purpose of training) and so gain experience prioritizing and working as a team. As the pretend patients get sicker, they transition back to the mannequins so no student victims have IVs started on them. Trauma is about moving people, according to Dave Carlbom, while at the same time taking care of them. So students drive around and talk to the dummy as if it were a real person.

A number of early medics who didn't retire on schedule during the last economic downturn now have finally done so, creating a shortage. King County applicants are given priority because it is in county bylaws that medics must be trained at Harborview. At the same time, class size is capped at twenty-four. Dr. Carlbom won't increase that number because "we are hand-crafting paramedics, not running them off an assembly line. Having more than that number of students in ten months would change the experience and not allow us to produce the excellent paramedics we hope to train."

The Harborview program still produces some of the best in the world. The EMS accreditation committee has called it a pre-hospital med school. The hope is to offer a bachelor's degree in paramedicine through the University of Washington.

As with any visionary change, however, this one came with some surprises: what happens when people who are really dead get intubated and shocked back to a heartbeat by the superbly trained paramedics?

8

SOME STAGES OF INSTABILITY

As well trained, industrious, and committed as they are, paramedics who provide pre-hospital care have limits; in the field, they lack all of the technical facilities available in a hospital. Since a pulse and inflating lungs no longer define a person who is alive, it is not uncommon for brain dead or otherwise unsalvageable patients to arrive in the ED assumed to be living. After sophisticated imaging, laboratory testing, and sequential physical examination and other evaluations, these dead patients can be identified. The trouble is, of course, there may be disagreements and misunderstanding.

By morning rounds at 6:00 a.m., almost everyone had heard about it. The newspaper ran the story on its front page in the morning edition, and it had been all over TV, radio, and the internet. The outrage wasn't even so much at what had happened to the car full of young people. At Harborview, they were used to that. It was about the driver of the other car.

A young man just arrived from abroad apparently had been causing his wealthy parents some trouble at home. An only child, at eighteen he was not in school and did not have a job. According to the papers, he was known to drink, drive too fast, and to have been arrested, though never locked up.

His parents had sent him to America to study in a Seattle community college, to which he was to travel from his condo in a new luxury vehicle. But he never actually started classes. He did register and met some potential classmates. A few days before the fall semester was to begin, he loaded three of these new friends into his new car and drove through town at seventy miles an hour, missing a stop sign.

With his foot still on the gas, he hit a car driven by a young woman who was taking her brother, sister, and a friend home. The impact was on the driver's side door of the other car. This was at a busy intersection near bars, restaurants, and shops still open late in the evening, so the police were there right away, along with Medic One. After figuring out where the gas line and electronics were from a computer diagram in their rig, the medics began to cut open the struck car with a blowtorch to get the passengers out. That took some time.

The other, brand-new vehicle was demolished, but the heavy frame protected those inside from any significant injuries. Because all the airbags deployed, no one in that car really got hurt. The driver and front-seat passenger didn't even get scratched, and the two in the back were only bruised. None of them had to be taken to the hospital.

The cops put the driver in the back of their patrol car and asked to see his license. He riffled through his wallet, telling them, "I have a license at home. Where I come from, I mean." They replied that that did not entitle him to drive in the United States. After reading him his rights, they told the young man that since he'd been involved in a serious accident resulting in major injuries, while driving without a valid license, they had to take him to jail, where he could post bond and be released in the morning.

"Maybe I can just give you the bond money right now," the young man said, still holding out his wallet. "Is $542 enough?"

The cops turned on their lights and took him downtown.

At the scene, the paramedics intubated three of the four from the other car. After she had a secure airway, they shocked the driver twice to restore her cardiac rhythm and pushed in 2,500 cc of IV fluid and drugs just to support her blood pressure. In the back of the rig on the way to Harborview, they had to shock her again. Her brother and sister were also intubated, although apparently less badly hurt, and the other passenger, a friend, was relatively stable. But by the time they all arrived at the HMC Emergency Department, the driver had blown her left pupil and wasn't moving the right side of her body, signs of a severe traumatic brain injury and pressure on her brainstem. One after another, all four of them went into one of the three dedicated Emergency Department CT scanners. Sandra Montoya, the twenty-one-year-old driver, was the most critical.

The CT scan of her brain showed contusions and clots on both sides, and her brainstem was badly compressed because of high pressure inside her skull. The scan of her body revealed the reason for her cardiac and vascular instability: a lacerated liver and spleen, blood in both her peritoneal and pleural cavities, probably a ruptured diaphragm. That much was ominous—more than ominous, really—but to give her every chance, the neurosurgery team put a bolt in her skull. ("Bolts" are plastic devices that are screwed into a patient's skull to hold a pressure monitor in place.)

The brother had a head injury, also seen on CT, though nothing like his older sister's, and the other sister had a pneumothorax that required the insertion of a chest tube in the ED. The relative in the car had long-bone fractures and abdominal injuries. Because they had injuries to multiple systems, these three all went straight to the Trauma ICU and looked like they would survive. Sandra, however, had probably lost her life on impact. Because the paramedics are so good at the job of rescue, sometimes people arrive at the ED ventilated and with a heartbeat but no chance of getting off life support. It takes a while to be sure of this, a time of desperate worry for families.

After the removal of her lacerated spleen, followed by a decompressive craniectomy, the last line of defense against a very swollen brain, Sandra went back to the TICU. The nurses covered her to the shoulders with a blanket so that the family members, who had quickly gathered around her bed, would not have to look at all the tubes: a Foley in her bladder, the arterial line, the IVs, the chest tubes, the central venous catheter. After several days of painful discussion and waning hope, the family agreed that the breathing tube should be removed. Their daughter never took a breath after that and soon arrested. Her parents donated their daughter's organs.

The other parents, the mother and father of the driver responsible, came to America and posted a $2 million bond for his release.[75]

Paramedics in the field, especially those in remote or geographically isolated areas, treat what they see in front of them, often with advice from a physician on the phone. They cannot possibly know all the details of an injury to a patient they are called to rescue, much less the subtleties of the beliefs and circumstances of his or her family. That does still require an emergency department, doctors, nurses, social workers, and sophisticated technology. So the medics try to save everyone. Their goal is to get each patient to a hospital, ventilated if necessary, and with a heartbeat, as fast as they possibly can. Sometimes this is by air rather than land.

9

AIRLIFT NORTHWEST

Airlift got its start in 1982 because of an electrical fire in a native cedar house near Sitka, Alaska. It happened that George Longenbaugh, the local general surgeon who had been on his own there for years, had organized a conference in landlocked Sitka, isolated on the western shore of Baranof Island facing the Gulf of Alaska. Mike Copass was one of the several speakers he imported to teach the local first responders about the emergency management of trauma.

The meeting was already underway at the time the fire broke out. Dr. Longenbaugh sat in the audience. By then he was already a vanishing sort of frontier surgeon, who did everything he could for his patients by himself, from gall bladder operations to diabetes control, usually without much equipment or backup. Before the founding of Airlift Northwest, sick and badly injured patients who had to be transferred to Seattle often went strapped to a stretcher occupying nine seats on an Alaska Airlines flight, crammed in along with medical equipment, nurse, and doctor. This solution was slow, inefficient, difficult, and expensive.

Occasionally before deciding what to do, Dr. Longenbaugh might bring a specialist up to Sitka, usually a fishing buddy, to see a patient. In the 1970s, when imaging was new, UW professor of neurological surgery Bill Kelly made several such flights to examine a hospitalized patient with a suspected neurological problem. If Longenbaugh could arrange it, such a long-range consultation could save a trip to Seattle for a patient who might not need to travel strapped to a board and, along with doctor, nurse, and gear, occupying nine airplane seats.

In a June 20, 2007 *Capital City Weekly* newspaper story written after Longenbaugh had died, his wife, Dee, said, "At that time we had a lot of logging around Sitka and that was a very dangerous job. Loggers would get hurt and they would bring them in by small plane. We had an old hospital, you'd just hope you could save them or get them out."[76]

Dr. Copass remembered going to eat lunch during a break in the conference,

and some old buzzard says "Hey doc, they're practicing your talk over at the hospital. There was a fire and a bunch of kids burned up." Just then, a waitress who was a little large for her garments answered the phone and hollered, "Is there a Dr. Kappas here? George needs you at the hospital. The fire department is sending a truck." A bright yellow fire truck came barreling around the corner. I got in and with alarm noticed that like so many vehicles in Alaska, the bottom was completely rusted out and you could see the ground rush past. So we go to the hospital and there was George hand ventilating one of the kids with an anesthesia machine, which I took over. There was a second kid over at the tiny Public Health Hospital, Mount Edgecumbe.[77]

Three children had been severely burned in the fire, and the only chance at saving anyone was to get them quickly to Seattle, so Copass called the Burn Center at HMC and was told to bring the survivors there. They all started looking for a plane and called every fixed-wing operator between Seattle and Sacramento. In the midst of that, Longenbaugh asked Copass to help him treat the two still-living children. By then, the third one had died. Longenbaugh, with his visitor first assisting, operated on one of the others, but before the plane arrived, that child succumbed to massive burns as well. The remaining girl had been resuscitated and had a blood pressure, so they thought she might tolerate the transport. "Pretty soon this jet showed up," Dr. Copass recalled, "and a smiling Jack got out with a gold medallion dangling around his neck, wearing a leather coat nicer than anything I'd even seen. So we loaded the girl up on a ventilator, with Janet Marvin and Lee Einfeldt, the HMC burn nurses who the plane had picked up at Boeing Field on the way, to take care of her en route. They wound up pumping on the poor kid's chest a lot of the way."

Janet Marvin, one of the flight nurses on that run, remembered the entire event:

On a Saturday morning just before Christmas, I received a call from Dr. Copass, or "uncle Mike" as some of us called him. He was in Sitka to lecture and there was a house fire involving three young girls each with greater than 70% burns. All were on ventilators. The hospital only had two ventilators so they were ventilating one child with an anesthesia machine. At the time we had been transporting burn patients using one of the Nordstrom planes when they were not flying the corporate people, but that day their plane was unavailable. So I began calling out-of-state flight services. After about three hours and multiple calls from the control tower in Sitka, I located a Lear Jet in Oregon, a plane that could accommodate 3 patients being ventilated and three staff members. The weather in Alaska was getting worse and the air traffic controller was getting anxious. We finally left about noon, but notified Dr. Copass when we got to the airport we found that the plane only had three E cylinders, or approximately enough oxygen for one patient for maybe an hour of the four hour flight. The tower said to proceed, that one patient had died and the hospital would send enough oxygen for the other patients. When we got to Sitka, we were told that a squall had just passed through and they needed to sweep the runway of hail and sleet. At this time we were getting low on fuel and diverted to Ketchikan to refuel. When we arrived, the airport office in Ketchikan was locked but the pilot knew how to find a key. We called an airport mechanic to come out to refuel the plane. The mechanic had to come in his own boat since the ferry had quit running. After refueling, the pilots said we would make one attempt, weather permitting, but if we could not land we would have to go into Juneau and spend the night. Approaching Sitka, the air traffic controller said there looked like there would be a slight break in the weather, and if we made a wide circle they could prepare the runway. We landed with a forty-five mile per hour cross wind to the runway, which is a landfill added to a small island off the coast of Sitka and had very large waves on either side of it. After we landed the control tower staff and half of Sitka burst in to applause. I have never been so scared. As we landed, the ambulance carrying the only surviving patient, Drs. Copass and Longenbaugh approached the runway. I got into the back of the ambulance because they were having trouble ventilating the patient and I suggested we do an escharotomy [the surgical removal of full thickness burned tissue] *on the chest wall to allow better ventilation. The EMT asked, "what do you need?" I said a scalpel and some 4X4's. He handed the scalpel to the surgeon, Dr. Longenbaugh, who handed to Dr. Copass, who handed it to me. So I did the escharotomy and they were able to ventilate her better. We moved the patient to the plane and prepared for takeoff. By this time the storm was getting worse. The pilot told the tower that when the wind speed got down to twenty-five miles per hour we would take off. We waited several minutes and the pilot said we could take off with winds at thirty miles per hour then at forty-five, he said. The tower then told us we'd be taking off at a very steep angle. So the flight home began. After about two and a half hours the patient coded, we began CPR and maintained the patient until we knew we were in American air space.*[78]

In fact, by the time they got over Dixon Inlet separating the Queen Charlottes and Southeast Alaska, the flight nurses informed the pilots that the child had died. The gold medallion captain hollered into the intercom, "Don't tell us that! That means legally we have to stop in Canada. Let us know when she dies the next time."[79]

Soon after they returned to Seattle, Copass cornered David Heinbach, then the director of the Burn Center, wondering about how to organize better transport, and he said, "If you have the time you can invent it."[80] Lying majestically about how much he already had to do, Dr. Copass told him that he had plenty of time to do that.

Janet Marvin had the idea that emergency transfer should involve just having to make one call to coordinate everything. That took some effort to organize, but thankfully Marvin and Copass had William Hall to help.

Hall, an army lieutenant colonel, had retired from Madigan to become a Children's Hospital administrator. He was a known force for getting things done and for always being firm but fair. In a September 16, 1994 obituary, Carol Beers wrote, "When the colonel drove to work, observers quipped, 'Here comes Col. Hall, wearing his Volkswagen.'"[81] The six-foot, four-inch administrator, who could lift men nearly his size off the ground with a single hug, didn't worry about image: Volkswagens ran well and saved you money.

A partnership between the University of Washington School of Medicine and three neighboring states with small populations and no medical schools, Alaska, Montana, and Idaho, had already been formed in 1971. Wyoming was added in 1996, creating the cooperation between all five Pacific Northwest states now known as WWAMI (pronounced *whammy*). The original goal was to help educate doctors for the Northwest region while encouraging them to return and practice in their home states. This plan provided some structure for the original Airlift operations in that cooperative alliances were already established so that medical professionals around the mountain west were familiar with one another and knew who to call for help.

Copass, Hall, and Ron Lemire, a UW faculty member for more than forty years and at the time medical director at Children's Hospital, went looking for systems that worked. St. Anthony's in Denver had one, but Copass felt "it seemed to be an employment program for retired Denver policemen. They had a helicopter stocked with kits in fishing tackle boxes for different problems so they needed minimal real time support, and a big communications center in the hospital." There was a program in Spokane that flew a respiratory therapist on each flight, which seemed a waste of manpower.

So the Seattle group decided to have a dedicated specialist RN for every problem they might have: obstetrics, cardiology, trauma, burns, and so on. Their training would be similar to the medic training, and they would be on call for the flights. But first they had to have a plane, and the hospital didn't want to buy one, though it was willing to invest in equipment. So the administration put out a request for proposals and selected Seattle Jet as the first vendor for Airlift. The company supplied the program with a Piper T-tailed Cheyenne 3.

The money to pay for transporting patients came from fees paid by insurance companies. There was an inter-hospital agreement in Seattle, which included all the hospitals except Swedish, agreeing that if the cost exceeded a patient's ability to pay above insurance, they all vowed to write it off. Before the WWAMI Region was formed, the initial goal was simply to get the patients out of Southeast Alaska on a fixed-wing plane and avoid the tragic delays of the Sitka fire.

To deliver babies and kids to Children's Hospital, they landed helicopters at Graves Field, the UW baseball field just west of Hec Edmondson Pavilion. While the original program included just the Cheyenne 3 fixed-wing, they soon started flying to the Olympic Peninsula, especially to Port Townsend. Airlift then approached the Army Medical Detachment based at Fort Lewis (now JBLM) about its existing program to retrain combat pilots for medical flights. By then, the army had been providing transport in several different forms for many years. Often personnel had moved rescue workers to sites on Mount Rainier, brought injured civilians off the mountain, and flown to and from other sites in Washington State. They responded to a fire department, or anyone else who called, so that they really functioned as an evacuation service. This was the MAST program: Military Assistance to Safety and Traffic. The arrangements were worked out with hospitals and supported by the army until the program ended in 1982. The law that had established the MAST program was then amended so that the military couldn't compete with private providers, and eventually MAST flights to help civilians ceased.

Today, Airlift Northwest provides much of the emergency evacuation of profoundly sick and injured people throughout the WWAMI Region. Former ER nurse and now Airlift director Chris Martin noted in a 2010 interview, "At Harborview we provided top-notch medical care to anyone, no matter what. At Airlift Northwest, we fly anyone, no matter what. Both are regional gems that shouldn't be taken for granted."[82]

Following the Oso landslide, which brought down an unstable mountain down onto a tiny community in the Cascade foothills, in April 2014, a story in the *Puget Sound Business Journal* noted,

Airlift Northwest's transport of 5 patients from the disaster was a reminder of the role played by the region's sole medical air service, which serves the critically ill and injured. The organization flies helicopters and planes, with about seventy-five medical staff, who care for patients in the air. It's staffed twenty-four hours a day, seven days a week. Airlift Northwest makes about 3,200 transports per year in its territory, which includes Washington, Alaska, Idaho and Montana. The organization operates on a forty million dollars per year budget and averages seven and a half million dollars in charity (unpaid) care. Although it's a nonprofit affiliated with the University of Washington, Airlift Northwest serves patients airlifted anywhere in this region, including to or from competing hospitals.[83]

One of the five badly injured people Airlift flew from the site of the huge Oso mudslide to Harborview was five-month-old Duke Suddarth, the youngest survivor. Paramedic Marty Ruffner's "ambulance crew was out on drill the morning of March 22, 2014, when they first picked up radio chatter about a landslide near the tiny northwest Washington town of Oso. Small landslides are not unusual in this forested rural area about 60 miles northeast of Seattle. The radio chirped with reports of downed power poles and lines and a barn that had slid into a road. Then it went silent. 'You really get suspicious when you don't hear anything,'" said Ruffner, who has twenty-five years of firefighting and paramedic experience. The City of Arlington Fire Department ambulance crew turned and headed toward the scene in anticipation that they might be needed. When they crested a hill on State Route 530 about four miles east of Oso, they saw this was no routine mudslide.

Ruffner was the first Advanced Life Support provider to arrive on the scene of what was the deadliest landslide in U.S. history, spanning one square mile and destroying forty-nine homes and other structures. "Both of my feet weren't even on the ground when somebody thrust a coat in my hands," Ruffner recalled. "I said, 'What's this?' He said, 'It's a patient.' Wrapped in the coat shielding him from the morning chill was a barely responsive baby boy with a large area of swelling on the back of his head. The patient, who would later come to be known to his caregivers as baby Duke, was one of very few rescued from the tragic scene in Oso and his experience underscores the value of training emergency responders and other healthcare providers in basic pediatric care."[84]

Baby Duke was operated upon acutely, and although he required more surgery, he eventually went home with his parents. But getting patients home isn't always so easy, especially when they are poor people transported to Harborview from elsewhere in the WWAMI Region.

It turns out that in many cases getting to the sick and injured in remote places is only the start of the story. One of the most curious unintended consequences of Airlift's success surfaced after a dysfunctional U.S. Congress finally passed a mangled form of the Patient Protection and Affordable Care Act first introduced in 2009, often abbreviated as Obama Care. As the Kaiser Family Foundation explained it,

> Under the Affordable Care Act (ACA), Medicaid plays a major role in covering more uninsured people. Most notably, the ACA expands Medicaid to nearly all low-income individuals under age 65 with incomes up to 138% federal poverty level (FPL), $16,105 per year for an individual in 2014. The June 2012 Supreme Court decision effectively made the Medicaid expansion an option. For states that implement the expansion, the federal government will finance 100% of the costs of those made newly eligible for Medicaid from 2014 to 2016 and then the federal contribution phases down to 90 percent by 2020 and beyond. States would continue to pay the traditional Medicaid match rate for increased participation among those currently eligible.[85] [emphasis added]

As a practical matter, however, and in part because Medicaid expansion is optional, the asymmetries between states in funding Medicaid have helped to promote various kinds of brokering for the better-insured patients. While this has, to some extent, always been the case, the search for the better insured has become more prevalent over the past few years. Skilled nursing facilities, adult family homes, long-term care and rehab facilities are more likely to accept patients with the best reimbursement schedules and reject those with Medicaid. After all, they are in business. So, for example, when a patient is now flown from Alaska to Harborview with a life-threatening injury and saved, and then requires either extensive rehabilitation or custodial care, there may be little monetary inducement for any of the available facilities in Alaska to repatriate that patient. Likewise, appropriate step-down facilities in Washington may be reluctant to accept an out-of-state Medicaid patient when they can fill that same bed with a Washington Medicaid resident or someone who has better commercial insurance. Since the number of these beds is finite, the result is often that patients who should either be returned to where they live, or at least be moved out of the only Level 1 Trauma Center in five states where beds are precious, cannot leave. The states in which these patients live aren't responsible for that bill—King County and Washington State taxpayers are. The costs involved for staffing, feeding, and caring for patients without medical indications or funding to be in an acute care center, but who remain hospitalized for sometimes months, are not modest.

These are problems that could not have been foreseen or even imagined when the altruistic founders of Airlift were first looking for efficient, rapid methods to move victims from rural areas to larger centers with appropriate facilities for taking care of them. For those doctors and flight nurses, all that mattered was saving the life of a sick patient. However, thirty-five years after the fire in Sitka that killed three children and initiated Airlift, there is now much more sophisticated testing and treatment to offer at places like Harborview, which are always over full.

Mike Copass directed Airlift NW until one night in 2008 after he himself had dull, aching chest pain that radiated into his left shoulder. In the event, he did not call 911. He called his pals at Seattle Medic One to come pick him up, saying, "Boys I need a ride." Then, with his wife walking behind, they haltingly made it up the flight of stairs to Avalon Drive and waited for the paramedics to come get him. They went straight to the University Hospital cath lab, where an angiogram revealed the occluded vessel in his heart, and then Copass was treated by the interventional cardiologist with a stent. He became a patient in the same healthcare system that he had helped manage, where he had treated thousands of patients and taught more thousands of medical students, paramedic students, and residents what it meant to be privileged to take care of sick people. Tolstoy said, "The biggest surprise in a man's life is old age." In this case, a fixture at the UW School of Medicine, the Harborview ED, Medic One, Airlift, the clinics, and the wards, indeed the City of Seattle, had been damaged, and it surprised both him and everyone else.

STATEWIDE EMERGENCY TRANSFER

One of the prime climbing destinations in the North Cascade Range is Liberty Bell massif near the eastern end of the North Cascades Highway. That is where Larry Deyo fell. On Saturday, August 4, 1984, the thirty-five-year-old dropped about 100 feet from just below the 7,800-foot summit and barely inside the Chelan County line.[86] Several of his climbing companions stayed with him while the rest descended and sped to the little town of Marblemount, where they reported to Okanogan County officials that their friend was injured and unable to walk. When told about this accident, William (Doc) Henry, the GP in Twisp, made ready to go help him.

The initial trouble was not in his getting there, or even how to get Deyo off the mountain, but rather a political barrier that grew into a dispute while the injured man lay on a mountaintop getting colder and colder. Of this episode Bill Henry later wrote in his book *Pay You in Hay: Tales from a Country Doctor*,

> *The medical and humanitarian aspects yield to the fact that each county sheriff has jurisdiction of all search and rescue activities in his county. This rescue presented us with a political challenge. The boundary between Okanogan County (our county) and Chelan County passes over Liberty Bell's highest point. The local sheriff's dispatcher was hesitant to order us to the rescue. The site was about 150 miles from the office and resources of the Chelan County sheriff, while we were about 28 miles away, equipped*

with supplies, ropes, and know-how. All afternoon we argued with two sheriffs' dispatchers citing the rapid approach of night and the reported severity of the injury.[87]

It wasn't until the next day that it was resolved. In the meantime, the climber, who had a badly fractured ankle, spent the night on top of Liberty Bell. He lost blood, the temperature fell to freezing, and there was no cover and scant remaining food. No water. What he did have was pain and fear.

Starting up the mountain at about 4:00 a.m. the following morning, a rescue team left from Twisp, reaching the injured man and his companions a few hours later just as a storm rolled in. They got an IV started and fluids running, stabilized him, and splinted the fractured foot. Bill Henry had managed to call Mike Copass, whom he had met during a prior wilderness rescue, who said he would accept the patient (a requirement for transport and admission) and dispatched Airlift Northwest.

Everyone left waiting on top of Liberty Bell was exposed to the elements and to hazard. According to Henry's account of the episode, all of them—including the injured climber—were struck by lightning, and several seriously injured. Miraculously, no one was killed. Doc Henry recalled their experience in his book: "Some felt as if the shock traveled from the peak to the clouds above, using their wet clothes as a lightning rod."[88]

After a flight of two hundred miles from Seattle, the Airlift pilot was able to identify a landing zone for the helicopter to put down near the stricken man and unload the flight nurses just as the lightning got worse.

The peak of Liberty Bell was windy, and the rotors of the chopper made things windier. Exposed to the elements and dodging persistent lightning, the crew loaded up the patient with one of the chopper's skids dangling off the summit. Bill and his EMT-trained daughter Cindy descended the winding, rutted mountain road and drove the ambulance back to his office at their new medical center building in Twisp.[89]

••••

Through the subalpine Cascade Mountains of Washington State, three valleys run northwest to southeast from the Canadian border. The central of these is the Methow, beginning along the Columbia at Pateros and ending west of Mazama on the way up to Washington Pass. Twisp, a native word meaning either yellowjacket or yellowjacket sting (depending on who you believe), is the valley's biggest town. These three valleys divide the state geographically and politically; like most places in America, there is a separation of thinking between the rural and urban regions. In Washington State, that divide is known as the "Cascade Curtain."

Before the North Cascades Highway 20 was built, these valleys and their sparse human inhabitants might as well have been on the other coast. There were few routes to get to them, and in winter, the passage to Twisp might be treacherous over either Snoqualmie or Stevens Passes, then north to where the Methow River empties into the Columbia at Pateros, then north again. Prior to the opening of the highway in 1972— arguably the most beautiful one-hundred-mile drive in the country—the Methow Valley was sparsely inhabited and stood alone, facing mountains on every side.

When Dr. William Henry arrived in this remote place with his family in 1960, he was already an experienced doctor, fully capable of caring for the routine ailments of the 750 potential patients then inhabiting the town of Twisp, plus those in the outlying region. However, he was on his own. There were no other physicians in town. No doctors closer than the small downriver town of Brewster, which in 1960 was home to only 940 people, but it did have a hospital. There were only 25,000 souls in the whole of Okanogan County at the time. When Doc Henry opened his practice, timber harvesting and sawmills still flourished, along with agriculture and cattle farming. The town had a few stores and more saloons. But in truth, it's tough for anyone to make a living in the Methow Valley, yet hardy folks still go on doing it.

In his book, Bill Henry recalled, "For as long as I can remember, it was taken for granted in my family that I would become a doctor." He was born in 1929 and grew up in Jennette, a small town in Pennsylvania, where his goals as a boy were "to own a car, and to go to medical school and be like Dr. Danny." Danny O'Connell was the local GP who made house calls all over the county and once sewed up young Bill Henry's lacerated forehead in the boy's own bed.[90]

Bill attended tiny Grove City College. While an undergrad, he met Ann Dwinelle, another Grove City student. They graduated in 1951 and were married two years later. Bill went to medical school at the University of Pittsburgh and then did an internship but not a residency, which at that time wasn't a requirement to enter general practice. These were the years of the Korean War, when most young doctors were likely to be drafted, as Bill Henry soon was. He went through the Navy School of Aviation Medicine in Pensacola, Florida, an environment that might have prepared him medically for his assignment to the Aleutian Islands in Alaska but did so in no other way.

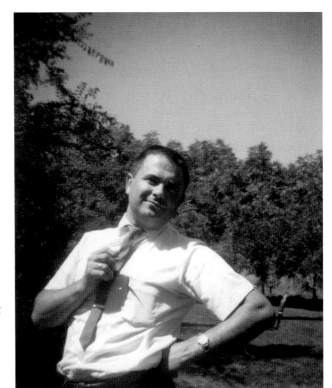

Right: Bill Henry, who always wore a white shirt and tie, early 1960s. *Courtesy of Cindy Henry Button.*

Below: Bill and Ann Henry with their children: Cindy pulling Bill in the wagon and Jane (who died while skiing) clinging to her mother's leg, summer 1963. *Courtesy of Cindy Henry Button.*

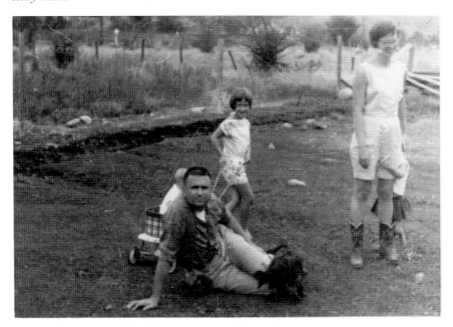

Henry was part of the search-and-rescue operations among the Aleut population who had been moved there when the Japanese threatened the island chain in World War II. He treated everything; he was all there was. Having never done it before, he successfully extracted an eleven-year-old boy's infected appendix, giving rise to what he called the "Henry Fake Factor," meaning when there is no alternative, you have to take what comes at you and do your best. "You fake it," he often said later.

When he finished his navy career at the Naval Air Station in Oak Harbor, Washington, he had two small children, a pregnant wife, no specialty training, and no job. He did have experience and confidence, however. In reality, during those years, he had been learning to be a country doctor, just like Dr. Danny.

A couple of navy friends from Eastern Washington encouraged Bill to replace the about-to-depart only GP in Twisp.[91] In November 1959, without a lot of information, Dr. and Mrs. Henry drove over Stevens Pass to arrive at what Ann remembers was a cold and gloomy little town. However, they both saw the possibilities for the kind of general practice and the life they were looking for, and with the encouragement of the bank president and other town fathers, Henry took the job.

"When I arrived," he wrote in his entertaining book, "hardly anyone noticed. I lived on the main street (which was four blocks long). I walked to work in the morning and then home again at lunch."[92] No one had much money to pay him, so within the first few months he had to borrow from the bank, but he did have plenty of work.

It was not always work he knew very well, however—like the time a couple of physician friends came to town to help him move into a house still full of unpacked boxes. While they all were hauling things out of the boxes and stacking them up, a longtime resident ran in yelling he was "snake bit." There are no rattlesnakes in Alaska, so Henry tried simply to calm the man while one of the young visiting doctors went into a back room and pulled out his copy of *Harrison's Textbook of Medicine* to read about snake antivenom. The patient "was on the examining table in the front room completely ignoring me because he was certain that this was his last day on earth."[93] It wasn't, though, because they successfully administered antivenom and drove the man to the closest hospital, where he recovered.

The closest hospital was at Brewster, almost fifty miles down the river. For the next thirty-five years, Doc Henry was to make rounds there at 6:00 a.m. and then go on to his office, where he treated patients from 9:00 to 5:00. In the thirty-five-bed Three Rivers hospital at Brewster, he operated

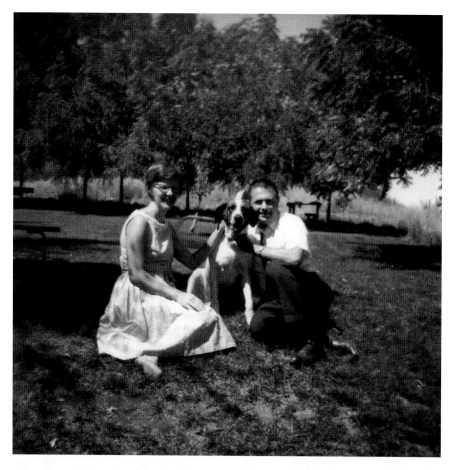

Ann and Bill Henry on the lawn of their rented house shortly after they arrived in Twisp. *Courtesy of Cindy Henry Button.*

on people for cholecystitis, hernias, appendicitis, exploratory laparotomy, C-sections and open fractures. He delivered babies there, in his office, and not infrequently in patient's homes. Several nights a week, he got up to drive out to see someone on a farm who was sick or afraid they were.

He started with an office nurse and then hired a receptionist. Ann paid the bills. They charged five dollars for an office call or nothing if the patient couldn't pay. In the 1970s, the rate tripled to a whopping fifteen dollars a visit.[94]

During these years, Bill Henry took on anything. "There is satisfaction in the versatility you are developing," he wrote. "You are becoming a master of many of the medical trades. This is balanced by the humble feeling that maybe you shouldn't be doing this—but who else can do it? Who else *will* do it? There are always the big city specialists, but these doctors are a hundred or more miles away. You are the best there is for these people. By accepting the challenge, you become better at it."[95]

Occasionally, he had a little help. His navy colleague Jim Baker joined him for two years, suddenly departing in 1969 to learn to become a smoke jumper so he could parachute into wildfires and treat people on site. How this worked out isn't well documented. The National Health Service Corps assigned a young doctor to Twisp briefly, but he didn't like it and also left. Every now and again Doc Henry was able to hire someone looking for adventure to do a brief *locum tenens* one hundred miles from other medical aid.

As he built his practice over the years, he also built an emergency house call bag full of the things commonly found in city hospitals. For certain problems, that was often enough, but more major trauma required transportation and Twisp didn't have any. So after having been forced for many years to rescue stranded or injured hunters, loggers, packers, smoke jumpers, and simply people lost in the surrounding mountain wilderness, Henry organized an ambulance company of about a dozen

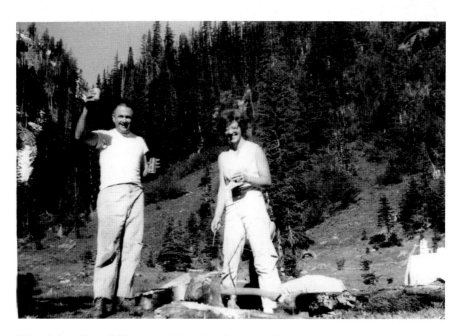

Bill and Ann Henry hiking in the Cascades. *Courtesy of Cindy Henry Button.*

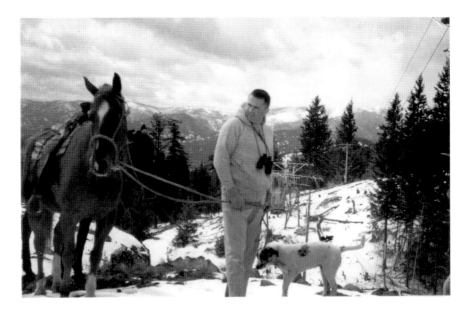

Doc Henry on a winter trip with LeRoy Gray. *Courtesy of Cindy Henry Button.*

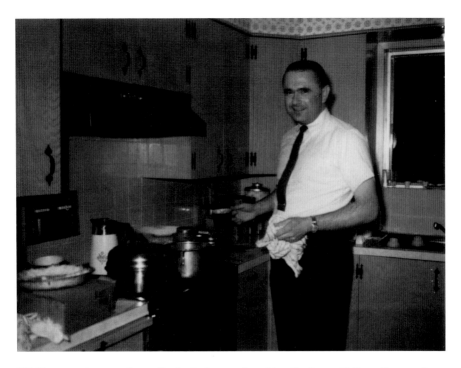

Bill Henry getting morning coffee in the house where his wife, Ann, still lives. *Courtesy of Cindy Henry Button.*

people. "The skills and techniques of the emergency medical technicians had not yet been defined," he wrote. "We created our own rules and protocols. We bought a Chevrolet Suburban, supplied it, equipped it, staffed it, and made it into an ambulance. Much of what we placed in the ambulance we scrounged, modified, or just simply made it ourselves. That homemade ambulance served us for twenty-six years."[96] He trained the staff himself, including his daughter Cindy Henry Button, who later became a paramedic.

Roy Farrell was president of the Washington chapter of the American College of Emergency Physicians in the mid-1970s and attended some of the EMS/Trauma System meetings with Bill. Farrell said, "He spoke about the EMS system he had created in the Methow. So on a subsequent trip, I stopped in to see him in his office in Twisp and we became friends. He asked me to come over and join him in his practice. I suggested instead that I come over for a month and give him a much-needed vacation."[97]

In September 1980, Farrell took a month off from his job in Seattle to allow Doc Henry a holiday, the longest he'd had in twenty years. For Roy, who worked in the orderly and well-managed Group Health system in Seattle, this month was an introduction to a world of some disorder and unscheduled obligation, including a twenty-five-mile run he took to Mazama to pick up a patient with a dangerous heart attack who was in second-degree heart block. Roy and his wife had gone with their five-month-old son up to Buttermilk Butte for an outing on a Sunday, "when the EMS radio on my belt went off. I raced down to town, got into the ambulance and we drove to the upper valley. I rode all the way down in the ambulance with the patient to the hospital in Brewster. By then he had stabilized, and I took care of him there, rather than sending him on to Wenatchee, returning home after dinner. Each day required a forty-minute drive to Brewster to make hospital rounds, then back to start seeing patients in the office. Some days I'd return to Brewster to make rounds on sick patients again and admit a new one or two."[98]

When Doc Henry returned, Dr. Farrell hadn't had more than four hours of uninterrupted sleep the whole month, and he was more than ready to go back to a more scheduled life. "Invariably, there were a couple of phone calls in the middle of the night. Occasionally, I had to go in to the office to take care of somebody with something that couldn't wait until morning. I told Bill that I would have more time to ski and climb in the Methow if I stayed in my job as an ED doc in Seattle than if I came to practice with him."

····

Bill Henry learned about better transportation out of the valley the first time Mike Copass showed up with Airlift in 1988. Copass knew and loved the Methow from his time working on farms and ranches there as a teenager and young man, and he knew at least something about the sparse medical care available there. The Okanogan County sheriff had contacted Airlift because a forty-three-year-old hiker had fallen in a stream in the Pasayten wilderness thirty miles from the trailhead and injured his knee so badly he couldn't walk out. He lay just off the trail between Hart's Pass and Loomis until a Forest Service crew spotted him six days later, by that time cold, out of food, and pretty sure he was going to die.[99] Copass directed the Airlift helicopter to the site himself, where the flight nurses picked up the injured man and took him briefly to the Twisp clinic, and then on to Seattle.

At the tiny medical center in Twisp, Doc Henry and Copass spent a little time together talking about the medical isolation of the central valley. Patients with serious injuries or illnesses often took hours to reach Wenatchee, Spokane, or Seattle, and in winter, it was sometimes difficult to move them anywhere. Henry and Copass were independent, tough, and industrious, just the sort of men who would like and admire each other. In addition, they had the experience of the Methow in common.

They met for the second time after the climber with the fractured ankle left at the top of Liberty Bell had been resuscitated, warmed up, stabilized, and the ankle splinted, when with some trepidation the Airlift team was able to ascend and fly the helicopter to Twisp, arriving at about the same moment Doc Henry and his daughter reached the small clinic. An office x-ray proved that the fracture was in good alignment but severe enough that an operation by an orthopedic trauma surgeon would be necessary. So they loaded the poor guy back into the helicopter and flew him to the chopper pad at Harborview, where he was taken straight to the operating room and fixed.[100]

All of these events convinced Drs. Henry and Copass to look for a better way to move such patients around the state. The Washington State Medical Association had organized a body originally called the EMS Advisory Committee to the Governor. This body survives in the Washington State Department of Health today as the exhaustingly named Emergency Medical Services and Trauma Care Steering Committee. Lothar Pinkers, a trauma surgeon from Bellevue, was an original member who helped to advise Governor Dan Evans. Jay Krantz from Swedish served, and so did Clyde Ballard, the owner of an ambulance company in Wenatchee who later became Speaker of the House in the Washington legislature. Bill Henry represented the practicing doctor from the boondocks.[101]

In October 1997, the Washington State Department of Health proposed an inquiry aimed at producing better, safer, and more equitable methods for moving acutely ill patients to bigger centers.[102]

This bill was created for the following reason: Emergency medical services and trauma care are provided to all residents of the state regardless of a person's ability to pay. Historically, hospitals and healthcare providers have been able to recover some of their financial losses incurred in caring for an uninsured or underinsured person by charging persons able to pay more. In recent years, the healthcare industry has undergone substantial changes. With the advent of managed health care programs and the adoption of new cost control measures, some hospitals and healthcare providers assert that it is difficult to shift costs for uninsured and underinsured patients onto insured patients.

The original committee met regularly in a room at the Ellensberg Holiday Inn, most remembered for its horrible red curtains, to discuss EMS, EMT, other first responders, and paramedics. Marvin Wayne, who supervised Whatcom Medic One medical operations, got involved. Dr. Wayne, also the state-appointed medical program director for all of Whatcom County at the time, directed the day-to-day medical operations of Whatcom Medic One. Under contract with the City of Bellingham, he also provided physician oversight for Western Washington University's paramedic training program and was an attending physician in the emergency department at St. Joseph Medical Center.[103]

As Copass recalled the early gatherings, "Lothar yelled, Marvin screamed, and Bill Henry, medically very sound and calm, was a voice of reason. Bill was rolling by the 1970s and was the force in the Central Valley. Aero Methow operated from Highway 21 that runs north–south through the Coleville Reservation to Washington Pass. That geography put them into conflict with Dr. Wayne, who considered himself in charge of everything into the Cascades."[104]

Marvin Wayne had taken a meandering course to Bellingham, a city north of Seattle near the Canadian line. He had first started a surgical residency, but when he quit, he was soon sent to Vietnam. Discharged, he moved to Seattle and began another surgery residency but again quit, thereby closing the chapter on his surgical aspirations. In 1974, he got a job at the St. Joseph's Hospital ED in Bellingham. There was already a primitive EMS system in place at St. Joe's, but ambulance service was poor. Wayne set out to create a Seattle-style Medic One he would direct. To get the trainees a field internship, he sent them to Harborview, and they soon began to provide service to the entire community. The same sorts of political problems plagued Dr. Wayne as they did the Seattle group, but Whatcom County Medic One grew in spite of it and is still taking injured skiers off Mount Baker with a helicopter that is part of Airlift.[105]

On one occasion, UW professor of medicine Len Hudson recalled encountering Dr. Wayne in the ED caring for an older man whose heart had stopped beating, and it "was clear to me that they weren't going to get this guy back because of age and duration of the arrest. Marvin wanted to open his chest. I said what are you doing?" Wayne answered, "We're saving this man's life, Doctor!"[106]

Growing up a lower-middle-class kid in Detroit, Marvin Wayne, like Michael Copass, had taken night and weekend jobs to pay his way through medical school. When Wayne was an undergrad, his father died of a heart attack at forty-seven, and a checkup revealed that the pudgy premed son also had, like Copass, markers for heart disease. And similar to Dr. Copass, he had a little bit of an edge, so the two of them didn't get along terribly well. But the committee on which they both served accomplished a great deal on behalf of sick and injured patients remote from major medical centers.

Eventually, the State of Washington did develop a plan that amalgamated counties into nine EMS & Trauma System Regions for implementing strategies and managing resources. This plan recognized the difference between rural and metropolitan fire departments and that "costs for pre-hospital services cover a vast array of participants and services." Lawmakers agreed that equipment and communications were essential in moving patients rapidly to major centers, and in 2003, the estimated cost of helicopter service alone could cost $1 million per year. At the same time, they established standards for education, licensing and certification for EMS personnel, and regional councils to oversee these activities.

This body, currently composed of about 30 members, is charged with advising the Department of Health of EMS and trauma care needs throughout the state. Specifically, the committee consists of representatives from surgeons and physicians, hospitals, prehospital providers, firefighters, local health departments, consumers, and other affected groups. The

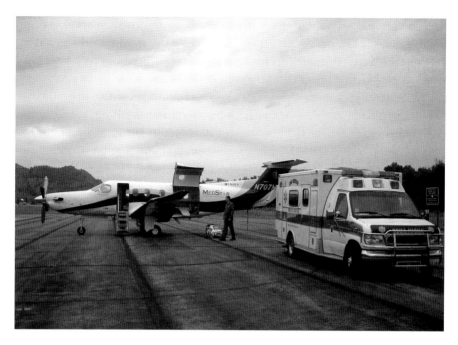

Aero Methow to Airlift NW transfer. *Courtesy of Aero Methow.*

committee also uses nine technical advisory committees (TACs) with more than 150 members from various disciplines. The steering committee provides guidance and direction to the state office in its development of the trauma system.[107]

Since 1968, Aero Methow, now directed by paramedic Cindy Button, Bill and Ann Henry's daughter, provides EMS services throughout the central valley, with a staff of twenty-six employees and volunteers. Their website notes they serve "2,000 square miles also extends westward into North Cascades National Park and north to the Canadian Border approximately 50 miles away. Though much of our service area lies within rugged wilderness where search and rescue resources are needed."[108] From its modern facility on Highway 20, Aero Methow employs a complement of eight vehicles, not including the snowmobiles, trail bikes, and rafts required for specialized mountain rescue winter and summer. Doc Henry would be pleased with the progress and probably more than a little surprised and relieved that, thanks to those local EMTs, Medic One, and Airlift, the HMC Level 1 Trauma Center is all a lot closer to rural counties than it was in 1960.

Bill Henry was a wonderful doctor, skilled, innovative, dedicated, and a faithful colleague to many. Roy Farrell wrote of him, "We remained friends until he died. He suffered a severe frontal lobe injury in a collision with another skier a few years after my month there and that really took a toll on him. Also, one of his daughters died while training for a ski race in Wenatchee. Ruptured her aorta when she slammed into a tree.[109]

AN ED REDACTED

G round and air pre-hospital management and evacuation weren't the only innovations in emergency medicine by the last decade of the twentieth century, and moments of extreme change are seldom placid. At the end of the nineteenth century, the great British neurologist and occasional aphorist John Hughlings Jackson remarked, "It takes fifty years to get a wrong idea out of medicine, and one hundred years to get a right one into medicine." While the timescale for modifications in what is now called the business of healthcare has dramatically shortened since then, Jackson's second-most famous observation, "He who was the first to abuse his fellow-man, instead of knocking out his brains without a word, laid thereby the basis of civilization," remains forever true.

The specialty of emergency medicine began its assent to board recognition in 1970, and like most ventures with vigorous partisans, there were many good reasons to promote that idea, some not so good, and a few that were simply self-serving. The American Academy of Emergency Medicine now remembers those events on its website:

> In 1970, the University Association for Emergency Medical Services (UAEMS) was formed for scientific and educational purposes by medical school faculty practicing emergency medicine. Prior to its establishment, medical students were already choosing emergency medicine as a career path. The first university emergency medicine residency arose at the University of Cincinnati in 1970. The Emergency Medicine Residents Association (EMRA) was formed in 1974 to unite the initial residents in our field.

The road to specialty recognition was particularly challenging. A provisional Section Council in emergency medicine was established in the AMA House of Delegates in 1973 and became permanent in 1975. Also in 1975, the Liaison Residency Endorsement Committee, the forerunner to the Residency Review Committee for Emergency Medicine (RRC/EM), was created. In 1976, the American Board of Emergency Medicine (ABEM) was incorporated, and the American Board of Medical Specialties (ABMS) finally recognized emergency medicine in 1979. Unlike the boards of other fields, ABEM was initially required to be conjoint with other medical specialties represented.[110]

While this drama unfolded, Dr. Kathleen Jobe, now associate professor of emergency medicine at UWMC, recalled that as a brand-new internal medicine resident, she had a bunch of pages from the hospital operator in quick succession one day. Standing in the Harborview Emergency Department that late summer morning she asked a nearby nurse a little irritably, "Who is this Copass guy who keeps paging me?"

"That would be me," came the answer from a few feet away.

Dr. Jobe, like most of the faculty who trained in those early years of pre-hospital care, believes that "Len Cobb had the idea for Medic One, and Vickery helped it get going, but Mike Copass built it."[111]

Among the younger people who had been trained in the University of Washington system, or worked there for years, this truth explains a certain cult of personality surrounding him. In the end, such an apotheosis might result in the problem of people believing any idea that came from someone they admired. When for whatever reasons the world of emergency medicine at HMC began to alter, Dr. Jobe said, "They didn't realize we were thirty years out of date."[112] There comes a time when forces demand evolution or extinction, no matter what systems might have worked in the past. In the heat of debate, a good bit of what is both claimed and denied on either side isn't true or doesn't matter. There aren't, in fact, a lot of things in medicine that stay absolutely true for very long.

But there are many ways to go about getting your way, and a variety of special interests supporting the new specialty of emergency medicine undertook campaigns both on behalf of the discipline and, regrettably it turned out, against individuals who seemed to be in the way of what they saw as progress at that moment.

Naturally, those involved in building the field supported the new specialty idea wherever they could, and many independent academic thinkers did too. But along those trenches dug into the ground floor at Harborview,

Dr. Copass didn't necessarily want doctors he hadn't selected and couldn't manage himself in his ER. He preferred to hire internists and surgeons of his own choosing and not be obligated to keep them around forever. As the tide slowly turned, the structures he had in place around him began to wash away. Since nothing had come easily to him, and because he had learned from his father that commitment to one's beliefs and to doing the right thing was a requirement—just as Benjamin Andrew Copass had preached and Dr. David Moore and his physician sons all believed—Mike Copass never backed away from a conflict of conviction.

In this case, however, he didn't realize that he'd lost before the argument had really begun. Late in the 1990s, young doctors being trained as emergency physicians did filter into the ED at Harborview, though this did not happen easily. On a posting board site titled the Student Doctor Network, which reviewed emergency medicine positions in 2005, unflattering comments still appear:

> *"Harborview Medical Center's Emergency Department, despite its stellar reputation for trauma care, has been ordered to hire emergency-medicine specialists or lose its national accreditation to train emergency doctors."*

> *"Harborview has no board-certified emergency-medicine physicians teaching newly minted resident doctors working for certification in the specialty, a violation of training standards."*

> *"Harborview promises to begin hiring the specialists. But the 34 emergency-medicine residents rotating through Harborview told deans at the affiliated University of Washington School of Medicine last week the plan is a 'superficial fix' and may force them to seek training elsewhere."*[113]

It wasn't simply young residents who complained. When trained emergency physicians, who after all had interests to protect, couldn't get their footing there, they too went public. In a February 10, 2005 *Seattle Times* article, staff medical writer Carol M. Ostrom, who had been contacted by a variety of people, reported:

> *"They've got the best of everything, except emergency medicine," said Dr. Ben Betteridge, a chief resident in the three-year training program. "The dirty little secret is there are no emergency-medicine trained doctors in the ER."*

"Harborview would appear to be the last place in the country that emergency-medicine residents are supervised on an emergency-department rotation by non-emergency-medicine-trained faculty," said Dr. Robert Suter, president of the American College of Emergency Physicians.

Harborview's plan is "woefully inadequate and unacceptable," said Dr. Richard Cummins, a UW professor and emergency-medicine specialist. He said it would continue to subject residents to a "substandard training experience."[114]

The dispute, which should have been settled quietly, employing the same evidence-based standards that are used throughout the rest of the medical profession to make decisions and promote improvements, instead became ad hominem, more than a little rancorous, and progressively more and more partisan. Moreover, at least in retrospect, the outcome was never in doubt.[115]

At the University of Washington Medical Center, Dr. Mickey Eisenberg, then the director of emergency medicine, seeing that the world was going in the direction of board certification for emergency department doctors, took some end runs at it. For example, he started an emergency medicine fellowship, but that turned out not to qualify people to sit for the boards and so was not a solution.

Finally, the dean appointed a committee to examine the question of whether or not to create a division of emergency medicine. It is certainly true that many, even most other medical schools, had switched to this model by then. While the committee decided not to recommend in favor of the plan, the dean had very little choice and did it anyhow, causing Dr. Copass to say about the program, "It's a mile wide and an inch deep." His vision remained that internists and surgeons should staff the ED, consulting other dedicated specialists when necessary. In fact, some argued, other emergency rooms around the state and the WWAMI Region were sending their sickest patients to Harborview exactly because they needed to be seen by specialists. But by then, not very many of those specialists really wanted a long career in the Harborview ED.

After a long, contentious negotiation, eight residents training in the relatively new specialty at Madigan Army Hospital joined four recently hired at UW on the Harborview rotations. As young army officers, the Madigan doctors were bold, ambitious, perhaps a little envious of the Harborview reputation, and certainly didn't like having been told they were unwelcome, the implication being they weren't good enough. Eventually, they were allowed into the trauma doc and Medic One doc positions. All of these young, therefore a little ungoverned and inexperienced residents, felt that they had nothing to learn from non-emergency medicine faculty, and it was their role to change the educational model of the Harborview Emergency Department. The first thing they ran into was the Hadrian's Wall of Michael K. Copass.

The Madigan residents arrived at Harborview when Kathy Jobe was the newly appointed emergency medicine residency director at UWMC. By then, Madigan had run a large program for several years, as training residents in this field suited the army's purposes. Very late that first year, the university got approval to begin training four emergency physicians. The result was that the initial group was made up of people who had had trouble matching elsewhere, a situation rectified the next year. Then the Residency Review Committee, a governing body, questioned why there were no trained emergency physicians supervising the ED residents, only physicians from the era of medicine and surgery attendings managing that population of patients.

That's when it blew up. The residents, not unreasonably, were worried that they wouldn't be allowed to take the exams required to become board certified, thereby becoming unemployable, and a few of their faculty and some of the Madigan attendings, who had careers to build, encouraged that thinking.

In order to practice medicine in the United States, doctors now have to be accredited by a specialty board, and a separate body, the ACGME (Accreditation Council for Graduate Medical Education), in turn governs those boards. The Residency Review Committee of the ACGME is charged with determining what programs comply with requirements for certification. In the brewing controversy over the Harborview Emergency Department, the battle was decided as soon as the ACGME threatened to withhold certification unless board-qualified emergency physicians trained the residents in the ED. No longer could doctors with other specialty board appointments, no matter how qualified or how long they had been doing it, be primarily accountable for the training of residents aimed at careers in emergency medicine.

The paramedics, nurses, doctors, and many of the administrators at Harborview, of course, supported Dr. Copass and his model, a system that had worked so well for so long, both locally and around the country. Along with HMC, the Harvard health system, the University of California at San Francisco, and others continued to use internists and surgeons to attend in their emergency departments for some time after the American Board of

Emergency Medicine was recognized, so that Dr. Robert Suter's comment about Harborview being the last such place in the country was one of many overstatements issued at the time.

Both Madigan and UW faculty members in emergency medicine began to talk in public and in the newspapers about what bad care patients were receiving. Dr. Jobe asserted, "It wasn't bad at all, but excellent; it was simply different than what they were used to."[116]

An example was the question of how best to treat tricyclic antidepressant ingestion. The HMC stance was that there was no good data to support charcoal decontamination for overdose, but that there were reasonable data supporting early gastric lavage. Inserting a nasogastric tube and flushing the drug out of the stomach was against the tide at the moment, and several doctors involved made their complaints about the practice publicly.[117] Not surprisingly, this became a focus of contention underscoring both of Dr. Jackson's quotes at the beginning of this chapter.

Some of the very doctors who supported the residents and their criticisms ironically had been trained and owed much of their success to Mike Copass, who had validated their claim that working under him counted as a fellowship. In some cases, that claim had been accepted, and therefore they were grandfathered into board eligibility without a formal residency in emergency medicine.

As the controversy deepened, a variety of people offered opinions about what had become an uncharacteristically public argument involving not only patient care but also medical education, including one judgment by someone who actually had firsthand experience. In an op-ed special to the *Seattle Times* on March 13, 2000, J. Michael Rona, then the president of Virginia Mason Medical Center, wrote about his years as a young Harborview administrator twenty-five years earlier. "Back then, a multitude of suburban hospitals were interested in becoming trauma centers," Rona remembered. There was debate "about the desire to become something and the difference between that and the ability to deliver on a promise." He pointed out that Harborview is the only hospital in the WWAMI Region with both the resources and the dedication to do that work, and ended by saying, "We are indeed lucky to have Harborview Medical Center as the level one trauma center in this region, and we are very fortunate to have Dr. Copass as its leader."[118]

A man forged by some hardship, who then found the structure of both medicine and the army stabilizing, Dr. Copass valued order and control. But he had never made a plan for his successors. To Dr. Jobe, this meant that "he had people working for him like me who could never stay around because of the academic promotion process. I was an acting instructor, which meant there was no track for advancement, so after four years I was out."[119] Copass himself wasn't necessarily thinking very far down that road; he was thinking about the patients in front of him.

Then in 2001, he had a heart attack. To many, the wonder was that it hadn't happened sooner.

By 2004, a group of five young Harborview doctors, Alice Brownstein, David Baker, Bob Kluse, Sam Warren, and Dave Carlbom, approached Copass and said, "You're aging, you've had an MI, you aren't slowing down as you said you would, and we want to apprentice under you so we can learn this leadership role." Around the hospital, this was called "the junta."[120]

Copass had been roughed up a little by the events surrounding the decision to bring emergency specialists into the Harborview ED. Long-held positions of authority are grudgingly relinquished, and the assertion of authority rather than its spontaneous acknowledgement required continued escalation, both on his part and on his behalf. He had, after all, pretty much invented the department, and Airlift, and a good bit of Medic One.

The philosopher Viktor Frankl said, "When we are no longer able to change a situation, we are challenged to change ourselves." For a person long in charge, evolution is difficult in the midst of conflict. Change requires a malleable way of seeing the world. While Mike Copass had many unique talents, adaptation was not among them. Initially, he felt they were trying to kick him out. But eventually, even he saw that change was inevitable, that the heart attack had changed him in the eyes of others, and that the doctors constituting the junta were really trying to help bring long-term stability and continuity to the only ED in Seattle and the WWAMI Region ready and able to take any patient.

The members of the junta had all seen Dr. Copass in the ED day and night for years, but that didn't really mean they knew all of what he was doing. To learn those things, they divided up the various jobs their teacher had helped to develop over more than thirty years and began to research Medic One, Airlift, medical education, and quality improvement. Under Alice Brownstein's direction, each day, one of the five became what they called the "E Com" or emergency communicator. They organized, put out fires, read the charts with Dr. Copass, and learned his codes: WTF, SEE ME, FAIR, and a new one, BBC (better by cab, in response to a question about the best mode of transport for a particular patient whom Copass knew to be a frequent ED patient). They also started to meet with hospital administrators to help quell disruption by rebuilding the schedules, talking to the residents, reassuring the nurses and the paramedics. Drs. Carlbom and Brownstein made the faculty ED schedule for the next five years, a duty that Dave Carlbom later said was "the hardest and most thankless thing I have ever done." Anyone ever tasked with making a schedule that involves more than one person will probably agree.

Harborview takes every patient who shows up, regardless of their illness or ability to pay, and through these years, they kept coming: people sick with pneumonia, heart failure, gonorrhea, blood sugars of more than 300, blood alcohol levels also of more than 300, gashes, infestations, and hypothermia from sleeping under a bridge in the winter. Medic One kept delivering patients found down, stabbed, shot, fractured, and comatose from traumatic brain injuries so severe that all that remained were their spinal reflexes. Airlift brought climbers who had been stranded or fallen in one of the mountain ranges. Even embattled, Dr. Copass still showed up to review the charts between 6:00 and 7:00 a.m., still insisted that all the patients be treated equally, and still clenched his jaw muscles or his glutes and looked off into space instead of directly at a person who had irritated him.

Both progressive sub-specialization and the competitive business models surrounding them have required county hospital EDs to be managed differently in the twenty-first century. There are few people anymore who are the database of medical information across many specialties that Mike Copass was himself and expected others to be. Fewer still will push in 500 mg of phenobarbital to halt seizures, turn the patient over, and intubate him themselves, then run down the hall to fetch a warm blanket. And there are none of them, no matter how dedicated, who will be able to keep an emergency department open without some patients with insurance good enough to help subsidize those with nothing.

Doctors often work in shifts and hand patients off to colleagues rather than assume complete responsibility for them throughout an illness. Residents' duty hours have limits now, and when they finish their training, they are often capable of caring for only a very specific set of problems. There are neurosurgeons, for example, who only operate on cerebral blood vessels, orthopedic surgeons who only operate on the pelvis, the knee, or the shoulder, internists who subspecialize in only certain diseases of lungs, kidneys, or hearts. Even those who train in family medicine are limited to the treatment of a relatively small range of common problems and seldom work on their own or even in small groups.

Professor of ethics and medicine Edmund Pellegrino defined profession as "greater than ordinary obligation." A few great American doctors have embodied that ideal, and to that list should be added the name of Michael Keys Copass, who put every patient before himself and whose mission in life was to treat each one perfectly while ensuring that all the young people who passed through his service became better doctors. In fact, that was the real basis of the controversy over what kind of specialists would attend in the Harborview Emergency Department. To the specialists in emergency medicine, it was an argument over turf, a view of the world in which they were better informed to manage whatever the paramedics pushed screaming through the electronically opened ED doors. To Copass, it was about who would care for the down and out, the mangled, the fractured, the psychotic, the terrified, the drunk, the filthy, and the infected—the unfortunates. Who would care for patients for whom no one else cared?

There may be more doctors like this in the future, but it will be a lot harder, and no one again will come in every morning at six o'clock for thirty-five years as Mike Copass did, or reach into a personal checking account to pay for the unfunded patients who wind up in a county hospital emergency department with terrible illness or injury and no money, as doctors belonging to county medical societies did in 1953.

Still, people in the hallways, cafeteria, offices, and conference rooms at Harborview don't talk about relative value units, income, or retirement plans. They don't worry much about who the patients are, where they come from, or what they do. They think more in terms of what's the illness here, how do I treat it best, how do I prevent complications or death, or where will this patient go from here when the acute illness is stable. How do I help this person who needs help?

And sometimes, when the heroic paramedics riding the Medic One rigs have preserved the heartbeat and respirations of a person who in reality was dead at the scene, they must ask how do I help this person to die in a way that the Bambuti Pygmies would recognize as dead forever.

The doctors, nurses, administrators, nursing assistants, custodians, technicians, and cafeteria workers at Harborview all think mainly about "The Mission," just as Mike Copass, Len Cobb, and Gordon Vickery expected them to.

After the heart attack, for the first time in his life Copass relaxed a little and began to spend more time with his children and grandchildren. Unwilling to evolve into something he couldn't agree with, in November 2008 he stepped down as the director of the Harborview Emergency Department. Then on December 15, 2013, he suffered a disabling stroke. Unable to continue as the EMS director, he retired completely, and Dr.

Michael Sayre assumed his role as the EMS fellowship director and medical director for the Seattle Fire Department.

When Mike Copass left the Harborview ED that he had largely built himself, the magazine *Seattle Business* ran a March 2009 story titled "Health Care Heroes":

> *All of medicine is composed of the fine balance between technical possibility and the desire to treat others as one hopes to be treated. It is this care of helpless, injured patients that perhaps requires the greatest expression of this responsibility. No one felt this requirement more deeply, tried harder to treat people with both technical mastery and humanistic reverence, and demanded the same diligence from all of those around him than Mike did.* [121]

12

THE DIGITAL FIREHOUSE

From the time the fire department began to organize Medic One in 1969, three problems have preoccupied managers and paramedics: how to get to where the patients are faster, how to improve their outcomes, and how to pay for those services in an equitable way. Technological developments in pre-hospital care have allowed firefighters to arrive at the scene earlier and with more to offer, and speed and outcomes are now much more easily measured.

Funding all of these activities has occasionally proven more contentious.

The arrival of the digital age in medicine transformed the ways in which patients are identified, treated, and recorded. When all of this information was written on paper, chart notes and data were difficult to aggregate into power sufficient to provide proof about what worked. The opinions of physicians, nurses, and managers were sometimes overvalued and often under certain. Dogma was of necessity based on accumulated experience and preconceived beliefs that might go back through several generations of teachers but had derived from small populations of patients often lumped together despite their differences. Because the experience of one valued instructor may be biased and prone to exaggeration as it gets repeated, such wisdom is now often dismissed as "eminence-based medicine."

Desktop computers have permitted aggregation of data into the meta-analysis of large, carefully chosen populations and produced the algorithms commonly referred to as "evidence-based." Like all information, decisions ultimately depend on the nature and quality of the data from which they

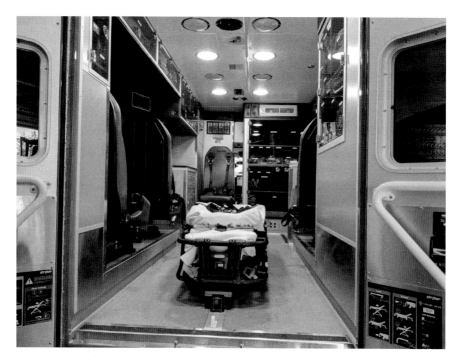

Inside modern Medic One rig. *Courtesy of Seattle Fire Department.*

are derived—beginning with its collection. In Washington State, that data gathering often starts with paramedics in the field.

The motto of King County Medic One is "Measure and Improve." That began with the original aid cars. Dr. Cobb and other Medic One investigators continue to foster this fundamental value of quality improvement to this day. More than fifty years ago, the *Seattle Times* reported, "Last year the department responded to 1,451 rescue emergencies, an average of about four a day." During that first year of operation, the paramedics riding Moby Pig marginally improved efforts to bring faster and more focused care to patients where they were found. By 1969, when Medic One was being set up, firefighters were responding to 5,096 medical cries for help, and that number has increased every year since. During all of that time, the reports filed by paramedics have been central in collecting the data that fuels the research leading to improvement.

The *Journal of the American Medical Association* reported that by 1972, dead people were routinely being resurrected in Seattle, just as Eldon Holmes was in February of that year. The *JAMA* article further noted,

[N]early 15,000 people in Seattle have been treated by Medic One since it was started in March 1970. Of that total, 36% were having some kind of "heart attack" when the unit arrived. The percentage of long-term survivors who were in ventricular fibrillation on arrival of Medic One has increased from 11% during the first 2 years to 25% in the past year [1973]. Medic One was one of the country's first mobile intensive coronary care systems. A number of them are in operation now, but no other city has such impressive survival statistics as Seattle.[122]

Over time, the matchless service provided by Medic One to local citizens has done nothing but get better. The Preface to the 2003 Annual Report to the King County Council outlined some of the key reasons for this success:

There are three themes in this year's report that I would like to highlight for the reader's attention, all related to the strength of partnership and collaboration. First, the continued strong collaboration between fire departments and paramedic providers, dispatch centers, physicians, hospitals, and the EMS Division is remarkably evident. This strong partnership is the cornerstone of the EMS system that the citizens of the county have depended on for over thirty years. This is manifested in a number of ways.

Thanks to the new method of integrating Seattle Fire Department data into the EMS Division database, we can now report easily on EMS activities across the entire county. We know that there were almost 148,000 EMS responses in 2002 and over 47,000 of these calls were acute enough to warrant a paramedic response. The equivalent of 9% of the population of King County is seen every year by EMS providers, however, the rate of increase in EMS calls is less than the rate in population growth, especially for paramedic responses. There is good evidence that our careful, appropriate changes in dispatch criteria have had a positive impact on managing the rate of growth in paramedic responses.[123]

By 2003, Seattle and King County had seven Medic One units providing emergency medical services to a population base of approximately 1.7 million people scattered over two thousand square miles. In addition to the cooperation that has characterized Seattle/King County Medic One and other fire districts, hospitals, and medical professionals since 1969, a variety of systems have been built to ensure the fastest, most appropriate, successful, and most equitable response to 911 calls. One of the most basic of these is the "two-tiered system."

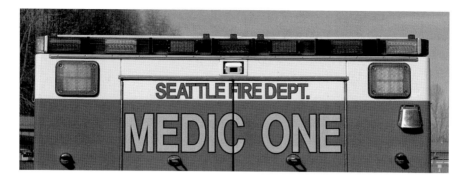

Medic One rig leaving fire house. *Courtesy of Seattle Fire Department.*

The EMS response system is tiered to ensure that 911 callers receive medical care dispensed by the most appropriate provider. Anyone can call 911 for help, but they might not know exactly what they need. Trained dispatchers triage these calls in six King County centers and, based on established criteria, then send either EMT firefighters educated in Basic Life Support (BLS, a requirement for employment in the fire department) or, in the case of immediately life-threatening conditions, send the second-tier Medic One rigs staffed by paramedics trained in Advanced Life Support (ALS). In 2003, about 30 percent of the total calls were answered by Medic One. Paramedics reached their destination in less than six minutes almost 82 percent of the time, and first-tier EMT responders were on site in fewer than fourteen minutes for nearly 96 percent of calls related mainly to cardiac or neurologic events, respiratory and abdominal illnesses, metabolic problems, or trauma.

In the same year, the efforts to improve data collection expanded with better methods and more jurisdictions involved. By December 2003, twelve agencies between Auburn and Shoreline and from Woodinville to Vashon Island were collecting EMS data electronically. Cardiac arrest was still a major reason for the dispatch of Medic One, accounting for about 30 percent of calls that year. Five-year survival rates for those patients successfully resuscitated by paramedics had improved from 39 percent in the 1976 to 1980 reporting period to 65 percent between 1996 and 2001.

One reason that King County Medic One has always been funded by a special levy rather than individual insurance is to guarantee that all citizens are protected. In an effort to measure whether or not access is truly universal, data concerning calls related to diabetes were measured in high- and low-poverty neighborhoods. Perhaps not surprisingly, more people in the disadvantaged neighborhoods called Medic One for diabetes-related health conditions because that was their best option. But in Seattle and King County, all these requests for help *are answered*.

In 2014, the last available reporting period, response times continued to reduce. Cardiac events still topped the mix of conditions reported, about 25 percent of them, followed by neurological illnesses, then respiratory, trauma, drug and alcohol, abdominal, metabolic, psychiatric, allergic, and obstetric problems. The great majority of calls involved patients between the ages of forty-five and eighty-four and peaked in the middle of the day.[124]

Again proving that Frank Pantridge, Len Cobb, and others in the 1960s were correct about the early treatment of cardiac events, in 2013 at least 62 percent of patients who suffered witnessed ventricular fibrillation survived to be discharged from the hospital. In fact, in Seattle a patient need not even have to wait for Medic One to arrive in order have a disorderly heart electrically adjusted. There are now more than 750 permanently installed Automated External Defibrillators (AED) scattered throughout the city, and a large portion of the population is trained in CPR. Dr. Michael Sayre, the Seattle Fire Department medical director, helped to expand this program even further by introducing "Pulse Point," a computer app to notify citizen volunteers in the region that there is a cardiac arrest near them. Using this technology, the Alarm Center can automatically contact people who have downloaded the app and have agreed to rush to give CPR when there is a cardiac event within a quarter mile of where they are. Dr. Sayre believes this might shave another minute off the response time it takes help to reach patients who have arrested.[125]

Likewise, advances in the treatment of stroke over the past decade now have increased survival statistics in regions with stroke centers, so long as patients are delivered to them promptly. In 2013, King County EMS transported 679 stroke victims fast enough so that 286 of them arrived within the four-hour treatment window.[126] The county also installed a stroke recognition program during this time, urging people to call for help when they suddenly developed signs of stroke. Again, according to Dr. Sayre, this system might be improved further. He hopes that before long, video cameras may be in place so dispatchers can see and virtually examine patients who might be having a stroke, providing greater sensitivity and accuracy of treatment.[127] In addition, new technologies are developing all the time that both broaden the window available for treating stroke victims and provide better methods for dissolving and/or removing clots that have formed inside cerebral blood vessels. The current management of ischemic strokes by stent-assisted clot recovery has proven effective.[128] In several large studies, patients treated by clot recovery within six hours of the onset of stroke symptoms employing a variety of systems, death and disability have been significantly reduced. In order to achieve these good results, of course, paramedics must get to the patients, stabilize them, and hurry to the nearest stroke center.

One area of concern for the fire department has essentially been eliminated because, while school fire drills remain mandatory, no fire-related deaths have occurred in King County schools since the 1950s. A frightening new category has been added, however—lockdown drills. Shooting deaths in schools, including some locally, have dramatically increased.

. . . .

In 2004, the Medic One Foundation established the Center for Pre-hospital Emergency Care under the direction of Dr. Graham Nichol. The foundation has endowed a chair named for Leonard Cobb, now occupied by Dr. Nichol, professor of medicine at UW.

In an effort to increase survival rates, the Center collaborates on studies with clinicians and researchers in a dozen countries. These investigations include evaluating the effects of early defibrillation, of bystander-initiated CPR, of the long-term outcomes following resuscitation, and of drug therapy required after successful resuscitation. Paramedics in the field have gathered much of the data that constitute the basis for these trials.[129]

Building on previously published studies, a potentially paradigm-changing paper Dr. Nichol and others published in the *New England Journal of Medicine* in 2015 challenged a longtime basic concept of CPR.[130] Since 1954, when James Elam and Peter Safar showed that expired air during mouth-to-mouth resuscitation was sufficient to maintain oxygenation, cardio-pulmonary resuscitation has included the breathing component. But beginning in 2008, studies began to appear suggesting that, at least in adults, simply compressing the chest produces enough circulation of already oxygenated blood to perfuse organs, including the brain, sufficient for effective metabolism at least for a while. In their randomized study of more than 23,000 patients, including 114 EMS reporting agencies, Nichol and coauthors compared patients treated with continuous chest compression to those treated by the traditional method of thirty compressions interrupted by two breaths, and found no statistical difference in survival or neurologic outcome.

Center for Pre-hospital Care–funded researchers are currently investigating topics that range from the evaluation of CT scans in patients who have survived "sudden death," better ways for 911 dispatchers to identify cardiac arrest and provide instruction by phone, and the prognosis for neurological recovery after cardiac arrest in patients treated with hypothermia. All of these efforts to improve responses to emergencies and to study the effects of treatments rely on data collected by paramedics.

For emergencies to be known, for EMTs and paramedics to be dispatched and arrive at the scene quickly, for data to be collected and lives to be saved, all of the activities of Medic One must be funded.

．．．．

The Boeing layoffs arrived in Seattle in 1970 at exactly the time Medic One did and produced a local unemployment rate of more than 10 percent. While the timing was terrible, somehow the combined efforts of Len Cobb, Gordon Vickery, local politicians, and, more than anything else, the citizens of Seattle found a way to pay for keeping people from dying. From the very beginning of the program, founders insisted that a special levy voted on every six years in King County should fund Medic One. They reasoned that such a tax regularly presented to the public would not only gauge the extent of Medic One support and value in the community but also ensure that every citizen had equal access to those life-saving services. While the levy has never failed, there have been obstructions.

Perhaps the greatest threat arose in late 1992 when, for reasons never entirely made plain, city council member Margaret Pageler, a fiscal conservative, and her staff took aim at Medic One funding. Not long after launching a campaign to redefine that funding into something more entrepreneurial, she had to go looking for damage control in a 1993 *Post-Intelligencer* opinion piece. Pageler laid out an argument that began "Budget crisis headlines fill this newspaper every day," and ended with, "The bottom line for me and my council colleagues is that the fire department must remain strong for both fighting fires and responding to medical emergencies. It would be reprehensible for the city to allow continued degradation of the department without looking for other resources."[131] In the several paragraphs between these two, she demonstrated a remarkable misunderstanding of politics, human nature, the Seattle Fire Department, firefighting in general, medical reimbursements, and emergency response. Pageler's argument that the fire department failed to collect potential private, as well as Medicare/Medicaid revenues, drew immediate contradiction from informed and influential people.

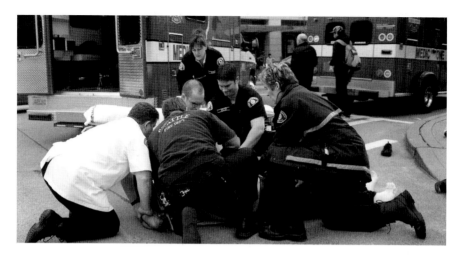

Modern paramedics at work. *Courtesy of Doug Bulger.*

On behalf of the Medic One Foundation, former Seattle fire chief Jack Richards and Dr. Cobb wrote in the November 11, 1992 *Seattle Times,*

> *We are particularly opposed to the proposal to instate a user fee, particularly since this program is paid for by city taxes and the King County–Seattle Emergency Medical System levy. At a time when the challenge of improving access to health care for all citizens is a prime topic of national and local political debate, it is important to realize that we in Seattle have achieved the goal of access for all citizens in the realm of emergency medical services.* [132]

Gordon Vickery didn't like the idea very much either and said so, nor did many other commentators both public and private. In the end, citing poor timing and fierce public opposition, Pageler dropped the idea.

A few years later, she applied for a job with the Greater Seattle Chamber of Commerce.

But Medic One persists and gets better every year. In 2015, the King County Council EMS Annual Report noted that both revenues and expenditures were increased. The levy rate for that year was 30.2 cents per $1,000 assessed valuation, meaning that the average homeowner pays only about $115 a year to fund the entire system. What do our citizens get for their money? The Annual Report tells us that now:

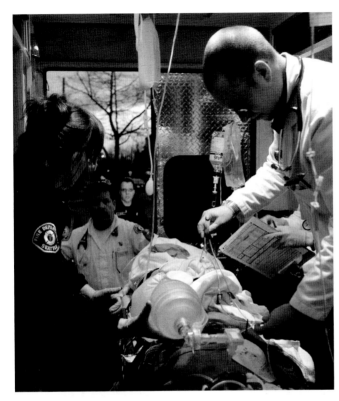

Left: Inside modern Medic One rig. *Courtesy of Doug Bulger.*

Below: Paramedic students (Ricky Gordon, closest, and others) take part in trauma training at Bellevue Fire Department training facility. *Courtesy of Medic One.*

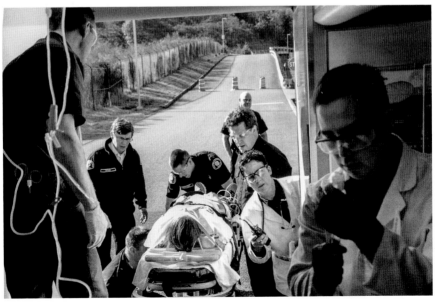

Medic One/Emergency Medical Services (EMS) serves nearly 2 million people in King County and provides life saving services on average every three minutes.

In 2014, firefighters responded to more than one hundred seventy-seven thousand calls in King County.

Paramedics responded to more than fifty thousand calls for advanced life support in King County. Compared to other cities, cardiac arrest victims are four to five times more likely to survive. This year one hundred-thirteen people in Seattle & King County were saved from cardiac arrest.[133]

Through the regular property tax special levy and contributions to the Medic One Foundation, all the citizens of Seattle and King County still have the same access to the lifesaving efforts of the Seattle/King County EMS system.

To restate Margaret Pageler, any other system would be reprehensible.

13

ALARM CENTER

At exactly twelve minutes and twenty seconds after eleven o'clock in the morning, a dispatcher at the Seattle Fire Alarm Center answered the call to 911 by pressing a computer key. For a few seconds, she listened, then calmly asked, "Is he awake and breathing normally?" A brief pause. "Where are you?" Pause. "We're on our way." She pushed a button on the screen that read, "*commit.*" The entire conversation from the time the dispatcher answered the call until she sent Medic One from the fire station closest to a child who had aspirated a Lego and was struggling to breathe lasted twenty-eight seconds. This is called the "call processing time" from phone pickup to dispatch, and until 2012, the average time was seventy-four seconds.

Since the introduction of a program called "Swift Dispatching," basic information about the location of the caller and nature of the problem is gathered electronically, and then, thanks to better technology, dispatchers can send help while getting the rest of the story. For certain kinds of illness, there is no reason to delay. If the dispatchers know something bad has happened—for example, if an elderly person taking blood thinners has fallen, has a head injury, and can't get up—that information alone is enough to dispatch the closest unit immediately. Often this time can be as fast as fifteen or twenty seconds. Depending on the urgency of the event and the distance to the closest fire station, since Swift Dispatching began, the average call processing time has declined to forty-seven seconds.[134]

A lot changed when Dick DeFaccio disarmed the fireboxes in 1975, and much more has happened since. The new Fire Alarm Center, located near Pioneer Square in Seattle, is physically part of Fire Station 10, a fenced sixty-three-thousand-square-foot complex that also houses the city's largest fire station and the fire department operations center. The building is modern, red on the bottom with a front façade of six traditional huge double doors that open to discharge the fire trucks. Above are several black metal rectangles that make a second story in various places. Long windows on these connected upper stories look like the slits in World War II gun emplacement bunkers.

The Alarm Center, a high school gym–sized room in one of the second-floor modules, is filled with flat screens and other electronic gear and staffed by trained dispatchers every hour of every day. In one corner, an electronic reader board lists the calls in process. All of the dispatchers are uniformed firefighters, and some are paramedics. Educated not only to collect and decipher information very quickly, they also have firsthand knowledge of the city and technical training in firefighting and emergency medicine.

The lights in the large room are dimmed to make the many screen stations more visible. Dispatchers wear headsets allowing them freedom to use both hands as they quickly populate the various fields that appear on the trio of computer screens at each workstation.

All the calls to 911 in Seattle initially arrive at the Seattle Police Department's West Precinct Station. That dispatcher first determines if the emergency is police or fire. When an injury has occurred and a crime is also involved, the police begin to interrogate that caller on the phone, while simultaneously connecting the fire department dispatcher to the call. If the issue is pure fire or EMS and no crime, the police dispatcher transfers the caller straight to fire. When both police and EMS are involved or potentially involved, then everyone stays on the line for a conference between cops, fire, and caller. The fire dispatchers coordinate with police to locate the place of the event, and if an assault has occurred, they try to ascertain the nature of the injuries. At this early stage, the conversation is fluid until the police collect enough details to know if the scene is secure and safe for the firefighters to enter.

The fire department dispatchers have a script that can take them in many directions depending on the problem facing a caller, and there are algorithms that include drop-down directions to guide them through any emergency. The room is calmly (but not coldly) efficient and resembles what one might imagine an airport flight control operation to look like in the evening. That is, business-like and intense.

Each computer is loaded with protocols detailing ways to manage everything from abdominal pain to Ebola infection. Of course, accidents of all kinds are covered, as well as assault, bleeding, trouble breathing, choking, convulsions, electrocution, falls, headache, poisoning, pregnancy and labor, psychiatric disturbances, and a universal category titled "sick unknown."

A fire dispatcher's first task is to locate the caller physically, if possible with an exact street address. If the call comes from a landline, they get that automatically, and the address is imported to the dispatch functions already loaded into the computer, so no time is lost or errors introduced in the transfer of information. But at least 70 percent of calls now arrive from cellphones, giving only the coordinates of the nearest cell tower. That's close, but not exact enough.

The largest barriers to collecting information are either an excited caller or someone who doesn't know where they are. If the former, then the dispatchers repeat the questions, speak in a calm tone of voice, and try to reassure the caller that help is on the way. When the problem is that the caller is lost, dispatchers advise them to ask someone else where they are, look at a

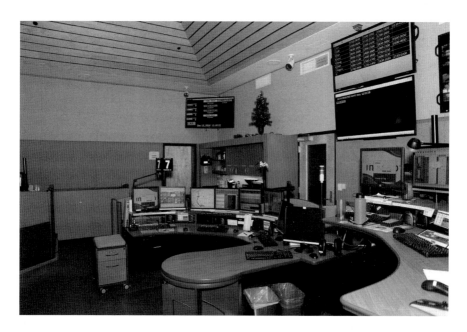

Digital alarm center workstation. *Courtesy of Seattle Fire Department.*

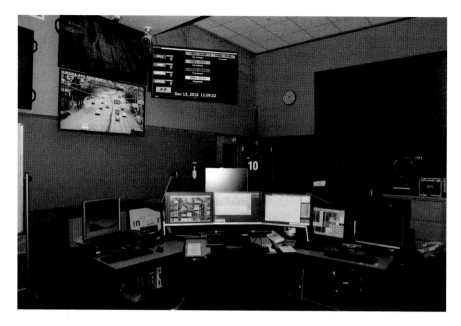

Digital alarm center console. *Courtesy of Seattle Fire Department.*

piece of mail, step outside and check the address and surroundings, or find a street sign. Freeways are the biggest challenge, but in that case, there are often multiple callers about the same emergency. Dispatch to a freeway is always to the location upstream from the event so that help can travel down the road in the correct direction. Because of the unknowns on freeways, the dispatchers are conservative about the time this might take.

The second two of the opening questions are also standard: is the patient conscious, and are they breathing normally. If either of these answers is no, after the closest firehouse is identified, Medic One is dispatched immediately. This can happen in as little as fifteen or twenty seconds.

The algorithms for each category of emergency are specific and designed to acquire as much information as fast as possible, while at the same time determining the level of need and the closest firehouse. For example, Protocol 11—*bleeding*—first asks the patient's age, what happened, where the blood is coming from, and whether it can be stopped by direct pressure. Next, they want to know if the blood is bright red (meaning it is likely arterial) and if it is vaginal whether or not the patient is pregnant. The dispatcher then determines the level of need, either EMS or the Advanced Life Support paramedics of Medic One. By this time, if the patient's location is known, the computer system already has determined the closest firehouse. If there is another fire or medical emergency going on simultaneously, the dispatcher can override the system's recommendation by handicapping both need and time in order not to deplete all the resources in that specific area of town. Then they press *commit*, the firefighters slide down the pole (these are still in use in many stations), the firehouse doors open, the lights flash, and the sirens scream. Help is coming.

But the dispatchers aren't necessarily finished. They continue talking to the caller and collect as much information as possible, data they can send to the rigs electronically while they are still en route. They are also able to offer advice for the few minutes until help arrives. The most vital, of course, is instruction on how to give CPR.

Paramedics continue to gather information at the scene, and Medic One physicians Len Cobb, Michael Sayre, and Graham Nichol follow up on the patient's hospital course and even their post-hospital outcomes.

In the field, medics have both enormous experience because of the intensive nature of their basic education, their always ongoing training, as well as a good deal of autonomy. However, if they require advice, there are still the Medic One and trauma docs available by cellphone in the radio room at Harborview, and Portable 55, now carried by Dr. Michael Sayre.

Jannett Wingett, a firefighter, paramedic, and quality assurance office for the Seattle Fire Department, notes that all of the procedures and outcomes of these efforts are under constant review. At monthly meetings, data are routinely reevaluated in efforts to make call processing faster and dispatch more efficient, as well as to update protocols and outcomes reviewed.[135]

Call center training is no longer an afterthought. Prior to the new Fire Station 10's opening in 2008, the education of dispatchers was not organized in the same way as paramedic training, and there wasn't a specific venue for instruction. Now there is a dedicated training room for dispatchers, adjacent to the actual call center where the equipment and arrangements mimic those computer systems and were designed for that purpose. It is also the backup center for police dispatch, which is backup for fire, so that in the event that one or the other of these sites is disabled, there is enough redundancy to keep going

In Seattle, there are approximately 430 cardiac arrests each year and, in King County, a total of about 700. Thanks to Medic One, 62 percent of these people now survive. Added to that are the falls, hemorrhages, strokes, seizures, crashes, the other traumas that befall human beings, all rescued by these same paramedics, who won't allow people to die at the scene. They won't let that happen because of their training, because of their commitment, and because of the doctors, nurses, and staff at Harborview and other hospitals of the mountain West who trust and rely upon them. They won't let someone die because of the extension of service provided by Airlift NW and the State Wide Emergency Transfer System. Perhaps most of all they won't let someone die because of the examples set by Len Cobb, Mike Copass, Gordon Vickery, and Doc Henry, still the heroes of Medic One who, beginning nearly fifty years ago, sought to build the most capable, fastest, dedicated, and inclusive system of pre-hospital care they could construct. That system is now matured, efficient, and successful.

14

EPILOGUE

J ust before noon on Thursday, September 24, 2015, the eight members of team two were standing inside room W251 of the Harborview Neuro Critical Care Unit discussing the occupant of that bed with her nurse. The patient, a fifty-eight-year old woman with a long history of hypertension, had bled from an aneurysm twelve days prior and then been operated upon the night of her admission. She was recovering well, eating, out of bed, and able to walk to the bathroom with stand-by help. The bedside nurse thought she might soon be fit to leave the unit. As the staff discussed her progress and plan for her continuing care, one of the assistant NCCU managers poked her head into the room and said, "There's been a big disaster downtown and we're getting survivors. We'll have to make room for them, so send anyone to the wards that can go as soon as possible. We've got maybe forty minutes."

One of the junior residents left and stepped to the nurses' station across the hall to look at bed availability. There he found a group of people gathered around a computer screen watching live feed from one of the Seattle TV Stations reporting from the scene. There was wreckage scattered along the Aurora Bridge connecting Ballard to Downtown Seattle and a "Ride the Ducks" vehicle slammed at 30 degrees into the side of a tour bus. The entire left side of the bus had been peeled off like a sardine can top. Bashed-in cars, debris, glass, fire engines, and Medic One rigs occupied both lanes of the bridge. About twenty Seattle firefighters were lined up beside the bus, a few more on the hood of the Duck, all of them carrying off people both dead and alive.

Because of the tag line that admitting residents enter into the electronic computer medical record briefly noting what befell each patient to land them in the hospital, this event became known at Harborview Medical Center as "Duck vs. Bus."

Forty-five minutes earlier, at 11:15, the Seattle Police had notified the Harborview Emergency Department about what they identified as a just occurred multiple-casualty incident. After the hospital operators sent out an implement External Disaster System announcement, the senior medical faculty members and managers immediately met to discuss a plan they had all practiced over and over for how to treat those patients they were sure to receive following such a catastrophe. Next, the hospital operators sent out another announcement to inform necessary staff that now the Internal Triage System had been implemented and that many casualties were soon to be expected. Following that second announcement, all the appropriate hospital staff assembled at predetermined positions to get ready. The Disaster Medical Control Center, which is the designation for Harborview medical control over the entire region in this situation, shifted into high gear.

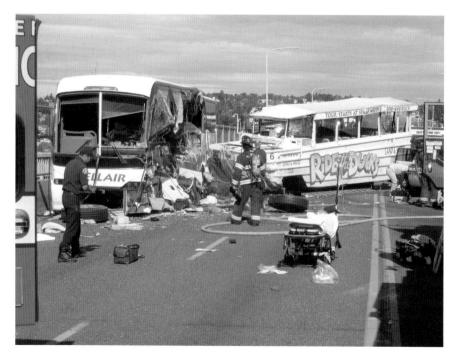

Ride the Ducks vehicle rams bus on Aurora Bridge at 11:15 a.m., September 24, 2015. *Courtesy of Seattle Fire Department.*

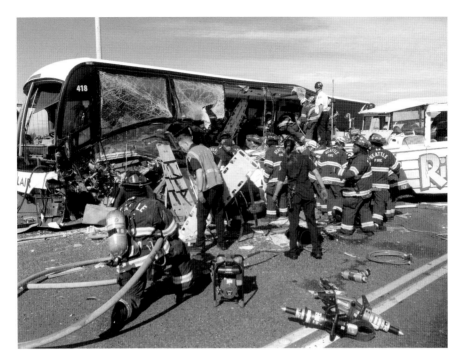

Firefighters remove the injured from crippled bus. *Courtesy of Seattle Fire Department.*

Because he was off that day, Dr. Steve Mitchell, director of the Emergency Department at Harborview, received these calls on his smart phone while working on a laptop in a Shoreline café. Although he left for the hospital immediately, several impediments required forty minutes for him to get there. It so happened that this crash, which involved mainly young Asian North Seattle College students on the tour bus, ironically occurred at the same time as an official visit to Seattle by Xi Jinping, president of the People's Republic of China. Preparations for that state occasion had already slowed traffic before the accident closed the Aurora Bridge, explaining Dr. Mitchell's delay, but the visit had also necessitated a staffing increase for Seattle Police and Firefighters. Whenever an important visitor is in town, two medic units are assigned to that detail, one for the principle and one for the motorcade. This is separate from all daily operations, and when the paramedics involved had finished their special responsibilities and returned to Harborview, they were already in gear and loaded to go. Also due to the staffing increase, several senior fire department leaders, including two battalion chiefs and a medical services officer, were already in the north end of town at a meeting. Since

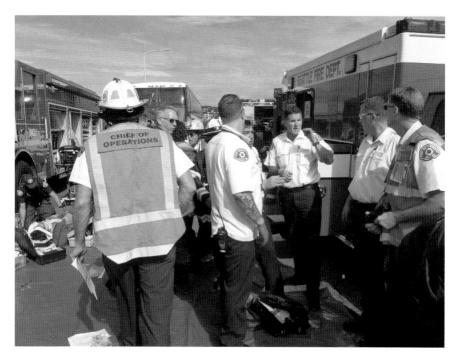

Firefighters prioritize hospital transfer from Aurora Bridge. *Courtesy of Seattle Fire Department.*

they were so close, those battalion chiefs were the first city officials on the scene. In the jargon of firefighters, they were the "first in."

Still earlier that morning at ten o'clock, thirty-six Ride the Duck Tour sightseeing passengers had climbed aboard one of the modified World War II–era army amphibious landing vehicles and left its downtown departure site near Seattle Center headed north to cross the Aurora Bridge. Just past Gasworks Park, the ten-ton Duck turned sharply and, for the passengers, a little unexpectedly to the right down a cement ramp and splashed noisily into Lake Union for the water part of the scheduled ninety-minute tour, always a surprising moment for visitors to Seattle. Returned to land and re-crossing the narrow Aurora Bridge headed back downtown, the Duck driver made his usual announcement that this was the passengers' best opportunity to photograph the lake. A sixty-one-year-old visitor from Florida stood up with his camera at the same time he heard the driver shout, "Oh no!"[136]

Ultimately, the National Transportation Safety Board reported their finding that the vehicle's front axle sheared off at that moment, causing the driver to lose control and swerve across traffic into the tour bus carrying the forty-five international students and staff. The likely cause, said the NTSB after completing its investigation a year later, was improper manufacturing and maintenance. These injured students, most having chosen to come to Seattle to improve their English, spoke a variety of other languages and were on a sightseeing tour before classes were scheduled to begin the following Monday.

By the time better information began to arrive in the radio room, that cubicle in the Harborview ED where the medical staff communicates directly with paramedics, fifty-one injured people were stretched out on colored tarps along the bridge. The four of them firefighters had put on the black tarp and covered their faces were dead.

Dr. Mitchell arrived at the Harborview ED about the same time as Medic One delivered the first of ultimately seventeen patients. He had begun his career as a fireman in 1983 and spent the last twelve years before he went to the UW Medical School as a Shoreline paramedic, so he had a firsthand understanding of the scene on the bridge. According to Steve Mitchell, "For decades the fire department had been practicing for multi-casualty incidents, and they believe that one reason for the great success in treating these patients so efficiently was because two Battalion Chiefs were almost immediately first in, so they were able to scale the scene and establish organization very quickly. They had control of access on both ends of the bridge, so they had two transportation corridors and crowd control."[137] The Engine Company at Fire Station 9 is only a little more than a mile from the north end of the bridge, Medic One #8 comes from Ballard, and Medic One #6 from the University District, but they were all part of the north end meeting and so arrived soon after the battalion chiefs. Both Mitchell and John Fisk, the MSO on the bridge that day, also believe that the way the department has simplified triage and early treatment plans helped insure very rapid transport of the injured patients to appropriate hospitals.[138]

The way that paramedics keep track of which patients have what kind of trauma is to stretch out the huge colored tarps at the scene of such an event. These code not necessarily the exact injury, but its urgency. Black means those people are already known to be dead. Red marks the most urgent still living patients and indicates that they have life-threatening injuries and must be moved to a Level I Trauma Center immediately. In Seattle and the WWAMI Region, red always means Harborview. Yellow indicates significant, but not major trauma, and green implies the walking wounded. Soon the trauma doc in the HMC radio room learned that at least ten "reds" were on the way.

One newly graduated paramedic, seen in news photos wearing his brand-new shirt, was on his first official run riding a Medic One rig, helped to resuscitate, and transported an intubated, sedated, and unstable patient. Suddenly, he smelled smoke. Something in the vehicle's engine had blown, and the rig stopped dead on James Street just before the I-5 freeway overpass where the road starts up a steep hill to Harborview, the same hill that had so often immobilized Moby Pig. The medics informed the Fire Alarm Center that the rig was disabled, and that they needed help. Immediately a nearby engine company and some police officers arrived just as the sedated patient's drugs wore off and she began to wake up—combative, thrashing around, and disoriented. While the others all held onto her and pulled the gurney out of the back of the rig, the more senior paramedic sent his new grad partner to gather drugs from the front so they could hold the patient still. All the while, the senior paramedic rhythmically squeezed the Ambu bag connected to that patient's endotracheal tube supplying oxygen to her lungs. As necessary as it may be, a large plastic tube in someone's throat isn't calming, so they paralyzed and sedated her with drugs. Then together the medics, firefighters, and cops all pushed patient, gurney, and gear up the giant incline to the ED entrance at Ninth and James.

The waiting triage staff wondered where in the world they had left the rig—and why.

While fire department and Harborview staff had trained for this sort of mass casualty event over many years, the biggest prior disaster involved not trauma but eight patients hospitalized in 2008 for carbon monoxide poisoning. Dr. Mitchell said later,

> This was a very different thing, but we were all ready, and it worked perfectly. The day-to-day clinical people who weren't necessarily specially trained for leadership roles, including the physician who took the radio room interface with medics, communicated with each other well, and both they and the paramedics stayed organized and efficient. Together they determined who should be transported to HMC and who could stay at a local community hospital. Initially, fifteen patients with major trauma came directly to Harborview, and two others were later transferred in from other hospitals when they were discovered to have more significant injuries than could have been known on the bridge. Within an hour and forty-one minutes from the time of the initial call to the Alarm Center until the last rig left the scene, Medic One transported all fifty-one patients. As a manager, I felt like a proud papa.[139]

Inside the ED, emergency physician Jeff Riddell was the trauma attending scheduled to work that shift and was already busy with the normal tasks of the day when the first call arrived from the Alarm Center. After the ED staff then huddled to establish priorities, one of them became the triage doctor and liaison, one stayed in the radio room as the trauma doc control for paramedics, and two others in addition to Dr. Riddell were each stationed in one of the four-bed trauma resuscitation rooms in the ED. They moved all the current patients out of the trauma bays onto the medicine side or into hallways. Then they set up ventilators and chest tubes by the beds in each resuscitation room just in case and called in extra nurses and respiratory therapists.[140]

The ED residents were still in a teaching conference, so their supervisor, Dr. Jamie Shandro, called to have all the most senior of them sent back. Together, she and the other attendings then decided that an emergency medicine doctor, a trauma surgeon, and an anesthesiologist would staff each of the three resuscitation rooms (each with four beds), so they had space for twelve patients at once. The three attendings stood in the middle of each resus room and stationed residents at the heads of the beds to help intubate, ventilate and put in the necessary arterial and venous lines, push in drugs and fluids, and stabilize the injured.[141]

When patients started rolling in, staff alternately assigned them to one of the three resus rooms, while calls kept coming overhead from the triage nurse saying, "We're getting more." In the radio room, the trauma doc had the TV on and could see real-time news images, so he knew what it looked like at the scene, but the rest of the ED people did not. Often the ED staff gets better information from news helicopters than from people on the ground, where things are more difficult to see in scale.

The first "red" patient to arrive was a twenty-year-old woman with a massive traumatic brain injury and severe facial fractures who had been intubated in field. Rapidly, the medics delivered patients with more head injuries, faces bashed in so severely they couldn't maintain a functional airway by the time they arrived and needed intubation, in addition to blunt abdominal trauma, vascular injuries, and multiple fractures.

After the triage nurse decided where each arriving patient should go, doctors in that room took sign out from paramedics. This involved a brief explanation of the mechanism of trauma, what injuries the medics knew about for sure, review of vital signs, and what treatments had already been given. But even the medics didn't know who had been on the Duck and who on the bus, or what exactly had happened in the event—what hit whom.

When a resident asked one of the medics what it was like on the bridge, he said, "Doc, it was chaos. There were bodies everywhere."

Gathering reliable information from the patients themselves was confounded by the fact that many of the survivors only spoke one of several different Asian languages and dialects. As a result, few people were even sure what language it was or who to call on the interpreter phone. One attending couldn't be certain if a patient looking at him blankly simply didn't comprehend or if he was having a subclinical seizure.

The doctors and nurses in the ED that day believe one of their most difficult tasks initially was moving patients to and from the ED radiology department. Everyone agreed from the beginning that all the patients sent to any one of the three CT scanners in the department would get the same scan from the top of their heads to mid-thigh. While this method might miss some extremity fractures, they would find almost everything else, and certainly all the life-threatening conditions could be known. Broken bones could wait. A neurosurgery resident was stationed at each scanner to identify urgent head injuries, blood clots that could require immediate surgical removal.

Dr. Ken Linnau, the ED radiology attending, arrived and took charge of coordinating who came next, where that patient was located, and how to return radiology reports to the attending in charge. Just the logistics of keeping track of so many badly injured people being moved around that quickly required vigilance. All of the records were being kept on paper because registration of the patients (most of whom could not immediately be clearly identified) and data entry into the electronic record system was too slow. Because identification was uncertain, the naming convention was also challenging. Ordinarily at HMC, if a patient's name and age can't be confirmed on admission, he or she is given the last name Doe, an arbitrary first name, and an age listed as 135 years until better information can be gathered. In this event, all the unknowns were listed with the surname "Disaster."

And since it really was about a disaster, crowd control had to be maintained. Everyone in the hospital knew what was happening and were intensely interested. The ED managers reminded people over the hospital PA system that it was equally important for everyone to take care of their routine daily tasks. In addition, the least ill patients in the five Harborview intensive care units still had to be moved to make room for the seventeen new casualties. To facilitate moving those patients able to leave the ICU, the regular medical and surgical wards had to put some patients due for discharge that day in the halls.

On that day, it happened that the hospital was full to bursting. All the ward and ICU beds were filled, and those hospitalized patients still waiting for beds occupied all the observation beds in the ED. In the ICUs, the nurse managers determined which patients were able to transfer out and then began to identify how many staff could be freed up to help in the ED. Nurses and managers in the Neuro Critical Care Unit discharged one patient to home, one patient to a skilled nursing facility, sent one patient who was awaiting a cardiac catheterization to the university cath lab, and transferred five patients to the floors. This took a huge coordinated effort that involved nurses, physicians, social workers, managers, and administrators from all areas of the hospital. In about an hour, the Neuro ICU had eight beds ready to accept critically injured patients.

And they were coming fast. In resuscitation room 2, all the beds were filled with patients who had suffered blunt trauma, and the staff had to intubate all four of them. Because they had an attending from each of the relevant specialties as well as a bunch of residents, they kept four teams busy, one for each patient bed, with the three attendings in the middle coordinating care. Trauma surgeon Sam Mandell said, "People stayed where they were assigned to be, so if beds 1 and 2 had patients for a while but the others didn't yet, the others stayed where they were supposed to be waiting, sort of like football players staying in their lanes."[142] Neurosurgery and ENT residents pushed a young woman from that room straight to the OR after a CT scan revealed a massive head injury and facial fractures. The first admitted "red" patient died in the Trauma ICU the next day, but before she did, the plastic surgeons did all they could to her face for the sake of her family. Sam Mandell operated on the young man transferred from Virginia Mason after an abdominal ultrasound there revealed free fluid in his peritoneal cavity, a finding that demanded immediate exploration of his abdomen. Dr. Mandell removed his lacerated spleen, and when he came to be seen in clinic a month later, he was well enough to return home to Indonesia.

During debriefing after the fact, most of the doctors and nurses mentioned the wonderful contributions made by the custodial staff in the ED that day. They turned the rooms around expertly and immediately: cleaned, decontaminated, emptied bins, and resupplied the rooms. At a major trauma center like Harborview, everyone has to pull hard on his own oar at the same time.

. . . .

In 1964, the Seattle Fire Department aid cars responded to about 4 medically related calls per day. In 2015, that number was nearly 150 calls each day. When Eileen Bulger, later to become professor of surgery, started out as a resident at Harborview in 1992, she had already had a career as a paramedic in Maryland before going to medical school. Steve Mitchell was still a paramedic in Shoreline then, and Dave Carlbom was a young volunteer firefighter on Bainbridge Island. All of these UW faculty members now help educate and manage the Western Washington Medic One paramedics. For all of these people, the motivations are simple: they want to prevent avoidable deaths.

As a resident, Dr. Bulger remembered, "I learned a lot from Mike Copass about how to care for people and do it with compassion. He put patients first in a chaotic environment, and everyone had to meet his standard. He was good at thinking on his feet with limited data. He was difficult when roused, but if you knew what he wanted and met expectations you did well."[143] She took over as ED director in 2008 for a few years because when Dr. Copass retired from that task he asked her to do it, and she couldn't say no to him.

Dr. Bulger and others have made the same effort to gather the data necessary to improve outcomes following trauma that Len Cobb initially collected regarding cardiac events. As one measure of the success of Medic One, a paper Dr. Bulger and others published in the *Journal of Emergency Medicine* in 2002 proved that successful pre-hospital endotracheal intubation by paramedics here was greater than 98 percent, the best in the country. Of this she said,

> Seattle-trained paramedics are always trying to improve themselves, and they see research as part of their job. When I got to the point of starting to do multicenter trials around the country, it became obvious that in many communities medics didn't see research as part of their job, and wanted to be paid extra to do it. Seattle medics wanted to do it because of the history of the program, and because of Mike Copass.[144]

A student in Paramedic Class 42 said,

> I was born & raised in the greater Seattle area. In school I enjoyed math and science, and I graduated from Western Washington University with a BS degree in Chemistry. During my senior year of college, I worked for a year as a lab technician in a large paper mill in Bellingham. The mill had an in-house emergency response team, and I witnessed their responses

to several medical and industrial accidents. This piqued my interest in emergency response. I started volunteering with a local fire department, and began testing to become a career firefighter. I have worked for the City of Bellevue Fire Department as a firefighter for 14 years. I applied for the King County Medic One program because I desire to be trained to the highest level possible, for the most frequent aspect of my job—seeing people that are in the midst of a medical emergency. I enjoy getting to build a relationship quickly with the citizens that call 911, and then provide them the appropriate immediate care. My goals are to obtain as much knowledge and experience as possible during the course of my training in the Medic One program. I want to continue to develop those skills in the field, learn from my peers, and pass on my desire and training to my future co-workers.[145]

All of the history, all of the effort since 1969, all of the lives saved after the Duck hit the bus in the Aurora Bridge crash, and all those yet to be saved, are summarized in the hopes of that young paramedic student.

If you have to have a heart attack or a severe injury, have it in Seattle, Western Washington, or the WWAMI Region, where—if you can be saved—Medic One or a paramedic trained by the UW–Harborview program will save you.

NOTES

Introduction

1. "Medical News," *JAMA* 229, no. 7 (August 12, 1974): 745–57.
2. "Professor Frank Pantridge" (obituary), *Telegraph* (London, UK), December 29, 2004, http://www.telegraph.co.uk/news/obituaries/1479924/Professor-Frank-Pantridge.html.
3. J.F. Pantridge and J.S. Geddes, "A Mobile Intensive Care Unit in the Management of Myocardia Infarction," *The Lancet* 290, no. 7510 (August 1967): 271–73; J.S. Geddes, A.A.J Adgey and J.F. Pantridge, "Prognosis after Recovery from Ventricular Fibrillation Complicating Ischaemic Heart-Disease," *The Lancet* 290, no. 7510 (August 1967): 273–75.
4. Emmett Watson, "Does the Name Vickery Ring a Bell? It Certainly Used To," *Seattle Times*, August 14, 1990, D-1.
5. Ann Henry and Cindy Button, interview with the author, February 18, 2015.

Chapter 1

6. Colin Turnbull, *The Forest People* (New York: Simon and Schuster, 1961).
7. Robert Leatha, and William Matthews, eds., *The Diary of Samuel Pepys*, vol. 1 (Berkeley: University of California Press, 1970), 1660.

8. Report of the Ad Hoc Committee of the Harvard Medical School to Examine the Definition of Brain Death, "A Definition of Irreversible Coma," *JAMA* 205, no. 6 (1968): 337–40.

9. H.H. Humphrey, "My Marathon Talk with Russia's Boss: Senator Humphrey Reports in Full on Khrushchev—His Threats, Jokes, Criticism of China's Communes," *Time, Inc.* (1959): 80–91.

10. M. Wallace, A. Yater, H. Traum, et al., "Coronary Artery Disease in Men Eighteen to Thirty-Nine Years of Age," *American Heart Journal* 36 (1948): 334–72.

Chapter 2

11. The details of Leonard Cobb's life and all the quotes attributed to him throughout the book are taken from his interviews with the author on May 5, 2015, and September 22, 2015.

12. The details of Gordon Vickery's life are taken from an interview with his son, A.D. Vickery, and the author on May 18, 2015.

13. Ibid.

14. Steve Miletich, "Firemen's Rescue Units Save Lives," *Seattle Times*, February 23, 1964.

15. "Mobile Coronary Care Unit," Seattle Fire Department newsletter 6, no. 35, September 5, 1969.

16. "City Gets Life Saving Cardiac Care Vehicle," *Seattle Times*, February 21, 1970.

17. Richard DeFaccio, interview with the author, June 17, 2015.

Chapter 3

18. Many of the details of his life and all quotes attributed to him throughout the book came from interviews conducted with Michael and Lucy Copass by the author on May 24, 2015, October 7, 2015, and May 20, 2016.

19. Many of the details of her childhood and all quotes attributed to Nancy Copass Tiederman came from an interview conducted with her by the author on November 21, 2015.

Chapter 4

20. Leonard Hudson, interview with the author, September 23, 2015.

21. Charles Russell, "Medic 1 Is Proving a Miracle on Wheels," *Seattle Post-Intelligencer*, May 1, 1970.

22. Bob Roberts, "A Case of Mickey Mouse Municipal Management," *KVI News/Commentary*, February 1, 1971.

23. "Heart to Heart Talk," *Seattle Post-Intelligencer*, September 25, 1970.

24. Details and quotes attributed to Wes Uhlman from an interview with the author on May 29, 2015.

25. Letter from Gordon Vickery to Bob Hardwick dated March 5, 1971, from A.D. Vickery collection.

26. Leonard Cobb, interview with the author, September 22, 2015.

27. Warren Young, "CPR—The Lifesaving Technique Everyone Should Know," *Reader's Digest* (January 1973).

28. Pat Fleet, interview with the author, August 5, 2015.

29. L.A. Cobb and H. Alvarez, "Three Years' Experience with a Pre-Hospital Emergency Care System in Seattle, Washington, USA," *World Health Organization Technical Report* Series No. 562, Annex 4, (1975): 110–14.

30. L.A. Cobb, R.S. Baum, H. Alvarez III, and W.A. Schaffer, "Resuscitation from Out-of-Hospital Ventricular Fibrillation: Four Year Follow-up," *Circulation* 52, suppl. III (1975): 223–28.

31. Professor Jennifer Adgey, letter to the author, November 28, 2015.

32. Leonard Hudson, interview with the author, September 23, 2015.

33. Editorial, "Medic One," *Seattle Post-Intelligencer*, October 2, 1974.

34. Herb Robinson, "Uhlman's Tinkering with Medic 1 Is a Political Enigma," *Seattle Times*, October 13, 1974.

35. "Uhlman Backs Down on Medic 1 Study," *Seattle Post-Intelligencer*, October 18, 1974.

36. Chris Martin, interviews with the author, May 21 and November 12, 2015.

37. Michael Oreskovich, interview with the author, April 8, 2015.

38. Ibid.

Chapter 5

39. Much of the detail and all of the quotes attributed to Richard DeFaccio are taken from his interviews with the author on April 20 and June 17, 2015.

40. Personal correspondence from Jerry Erhler to the author dated December 3, 2015.
41. Ibid.

Chapter 6

42. "Accidental Death and Disability: the Neglected Diseases of Modern Society," *Division of Medical Sciences, National Academy of Sciences, National Research Council. Washington, DC* (1966).
43. Jackson Déziel, "Past Medical History: Paramedics in the United States" (unpublished undergraduate thesis, Western Carolina University, 2006).
44. Manish Shah, "The Formation of the Emergency Medical Services System," *Am. J. Public Health* 96, no. 3 (2006): 414–23.
45. James O. Page Papers Manuscript Collection no. 461, History & Special Collections for the Sciences, Louise M. Darling Biomedical Library, UCLA.
46. Ibid.
47. Déziel, "Past Medical History."
48. Los Angeles Emergency Medical Services (EMS) Agency, http://dhs. lacounty.gov/wps/portal/dhs/ems.
49. D. Davis, M. Ochs, D. Hoyt, et al., "The San Diego Paramedic Rapid Sequence Intubation Trial: A Three Year Experience," *Academic Emergency Medicine* 10, no 5 (2003): 446.
50. James Page, *The Paramedics: An Illustrated History of Paramedics in Their First Decade in the USA* (Morristown, NJ: Backdraft Publications, 1979).
51. Ibid.
52. US Patent Office Publication Number 1371702 A: (March 15, 1921).
53. J. Warren, F. Hill, and L. Faehnie, *The Columbus Story of Mobile Emergency Care*, Ohio State University Department of Medicine pamphlet, 1975.
54. Déziel, "Past Medical History."
55. "How Pittsburgh's Freedom House Pioneered Paramedic Treatment," *All Things Considered*, March 21, 2015.
56. Ibid.
57. Chuck Staresinic, "Send Freedom House," *Pitt Med Magazine* (February 2004).
58. Wikipedia, "Peter Safar," https://en.wikipedia.org/wiki/Peter_Safar.
59. Staresinic, "Send Freedom House."
60. Ibid.

61. Pittsburgh Emergency Medical Services, http://pittsburghpa.gov/ems.

62. Eugene L. Nagel, MD Collection: Finding Aid, Wood Library-Museum of Anesthesiology, Park Ridge, IL, November 26, 2012.

63. Mickey Eisenberg, MD, PhD, *Life in the Balance* (Oxford, UK: Oxford University Press, 1997).

64. M. Eisenberg, "Eugene Nagel and the Miami Paramedic Program." *Resuscitation* 56: (2003): 243–46.

65. Eisenberg, *Life in the Balance*.

66. Eisenberg, "Eugene Nagel," 243–46.

67. James O. Page Papers Manuscript Collection no. 461, History & Special Collections for the Sciences, Louise M. Darling Biomedical Library, UCLA.

68. Eisenberg, *Life in the Balance*.

69. Fire-Rescue Department—City of Miami, https://www.miamigov.com/Government/Departments-Organizations/Fire-Rescue.

70. U.S. Bureau of Labor Statistics, https://www.bls.gov.

Chapter 7

71. David Carlbom, interview with the author, August 10, 2015.

72. Ibid.

73. Ibid.

74. Ibid.

Chapter 8

75. Sara Jean Green, "Chinese Student Convicted of Fatal Des Moines Crash Deported," *Seattle Times*, November 21, 2014.

Chapter 9

76. Weld Royal, "Airlift Northwest Helping Southeast Alaskans with Medical Assistance for the Past 25 Years," *Capital City Weekly* (2007).

77. Interviews conducted by the author with Michael and Lucy Copass on May 24, 2015, October 7, 2015, and May 20, 2016.

78. Janet Marvin, e-mail to the author on December 5, 2015.

79. Copass, interviews.

80. Ibid.

81. Carole Beers, "William Hall, A Firm but Fair Leader, Hospital Administrator," *Seattle Times*, September 16, 1994.

82. Chris Martin, interviews with the author on May 21 and November 12, 2015.

83. Valerie Bauman, "The Most Important Flight You'd Ever Take: Airlift Northwest," *Puget Sound Business Journal*, April 27, 2014, http://www.bizjournals.com/seattle/blog/health-care-inc/2014/04/ost-important-flight-youd-ever-take-airlift.html.

84. Jessica Brown and Kirk Boxleitner, "Baby Duke Still in Recovery," *Arlington Times*, March 5, 2016.

85. Robin Rudowitz, "Understanding How States Access the ACA Enhanced Medicaid Match Rates," The Henry J. Kaiser Family Foundation, September 29, 2014, http://kff.org/medicaid/issue-brief/understanding-how-states-access-the-aca-enhanced-medicaid-match-rates.

Chapter 10

86. Delores Riggs, "Lightening Makes for Harrowing Rescue," *Wenatchee World*, 1984.

87. William Henry, *Pay You in Hay* (Gig Harbor, WA: Red Apple Publishing, 1999).

88. Ibid.

89. Ann Henry and Cindy Button, interview with the author, February 18, 2015.

90. Henry, *Pay You in Hay*.

91. Button, interview.

92. Henry, *Pay You in Hay*.

93. Ibid.

94. Button, interview.

95. Henry, *Pay You in Hay*.

96. Ibid.

97. Roy Farrell, interview with the author, June 7, 2015.

98. Ibid.

99. Patricia Wren, "Injured, Alone, Man Survives for Six Days," *Wenatchee World, Okanogan County Bureau*, September 1, 1988.

100. Button, interview.

101. Michael and Lucy Copass, interviews with the author, May 24, 2015, October 7, 2015, and May 20, 2016.

102. WRR 97-21-136 Filed October 22, 1997, 9:21 a.m., http://lawfilesext. leg.wa.gov/law/wsr/1997/21/97-21-136.htm.

103. Marvin Wayne, interview with the author, August 26, 2015.

104. Copass, interviews.

105. Wayne, interview.

106. Leonard Hudson, interview with the author, September 23, 2015.

107. Emergency Medical Services (EMS) Systems, http://www.doh.wa.gov/ ForPublicHealthandHealthcareProviders/EmergencyMedical ServicesEMSSystems/EMSandTrauma/CouncilsandCommittees/ EMSandTraumaSteeringCommittee.

108. Aero Methow, http://www.aeromethow.org.

109. Roy Farrell, interview with the author, June 7, 2015.

Chapter 11

110. American Academy of Emergency Medicine, http://www.aaem.org/ about-aaem/aaem-history.

111. Kathleen Jobe, interview with the author, September 18, 2015.

112. Ibid.

113. Madigan Army Medical Center (U Washington) Residency Reviews, http://forums.studentdoctor.net/threads/madigan-army-medical-center-u-washington-residency-reviews.770550.

114. Carol Ostrom, "Clash Over ER Training Could Hurt Harborview," *Seattle Times*, February 10, 2005, http://www.seattletimes.com/seattle-news/clash-over-er-training-could-hurt-harborview.

115. Ibid.

116. Jobe, interview.

117. Carol Ostrom, personal correspondence with the author, October 23, 2015.

118. J. Michael Rona, "Politics of a World Class Trauma Center," *Seattle Times*, March 13, 2000.

119. Jobe, interview.

120. David Carlbom, interview with the author, August 10, 2015.

121. Dean Paton, "Health Care Heroes 2009," *Seattle Business* (March 2009), http://www.seattlebusinessmag.com/article/health-care-heroes-2009?page=0,2.

Chapter 12

122. "Medical News," *JAMA* 229, no. 7 (August 12, 1974): 745–57.

123. King County Reports and Publications, http://www.kingcounty.gov/healthservices/health/ems/reports.aspx.

124. A.C. Leung, D.A. Asch, K.N. Lozada, "Where Are Lifesaving Automated External Defibrillators Located and How Hard Is It to Find Them in a Large Urban City?," *Resuscitation* 84, no. 7 (2013): 910–14, https://www.ncbi.nlm.nih.gov/pubmed/23357702.

125. Michael Sayre, interview with the author, January 11, 2016.

126. Ibid.

127. Ibid.

128. J.E. Cohen, J.M. Gomori, R.R. Leker, et al., "Recanalization with Stent-Based Mechanical Thrombectomy in Anterior Circulation Major Ischemic Stroke," *J Clin Neuroscience* 19 (2012): 39–43.

129. Graham Nichol, interview with the author, January 18, 2016.

130. G. Nichol, B. Leroux, H. Wang, et al., "Trial of Continuous Chest Compressions During CPR," *New England Journal of Medicine* 373: (2015): 2203–14.

131. Margaret Pageler, "More Resources Needed to Pay for Medic 1 Emergency Services," *Seattle Post-Intelligencer*, March 2, 1993.

132. L. Cobb and J. Richards, "Charging for Medic One Would Undermine Service," *Seattle Times*, November 11, 1992.

133. King County Reports and Publications, http://www.kingcounty.gov/healthservices/health/ems/reports.aspx.

Chapter 13

134. Janett Wingett, interview with the author, December 21, 2015.

135. Ibid.

Chapter 14

136. Seattle Times Staff, "12 Seriously Injured in Crash on Aurora Bridge," *Seattle Times*, September 25, 2015.

137. Steven Mitchell, interview with the author, November 17, 2015.

138. John Fisk, interview with the author, January 7, 2016.

139. Mitchell, interview.

140. Jeff Riddell, interview with the author, November 4, 2015.

141. Jamie Shandro, interview with the author, November 11, 2015.

142. Sam Mandell, interview with the author, November 13, 2015.

143. Eileen Bulger, interview with the author, November 12, 2015.

144. E. Bulger, M. Copass, R. Maier, et al, "An Analysis of Advanced Pre-hospital Airway Management," *Journal of Emergency Medicine* 23, no. 2: (2002): 183–89.

145. Scott Symons, letter to the author, December 10, 2015.

INDEX

ABOUT THE AUTHOR

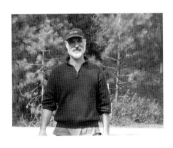

R ichard Rapport is a clinical professor at the University of Washington School of Medicine in both the Department of Neurological Surgery and the Department of Global Health. He is the author of *PHYSICIAN: The Life of Paul Beeson* (nominated for the Washington State Book Award) and *NERVE Endings: The Discovery of the Synapse* (nominated for the Washington State Book Award and the Aventis Prize). He has published dozens of professional papers, as well as essays in journals and literary magazines, including *The American Scholar*, *The Pharos*, *Poetry*, *The Northwest Review*, *Seattle Review*, *Open Spaces*, and *The Threepenny Review*. Two of these essays were nominated for the Pushcart Prize, and one was noted in *Best American Essays*.

Dr. Rapport is an attending physician at Harborview Medical Center in Seattle, where among other duties he is the co-site director for the UW medical students' neurosurgical elective course. He is married to the writer Valerie Trueblood.